HAPPY SACHI'S YOGA

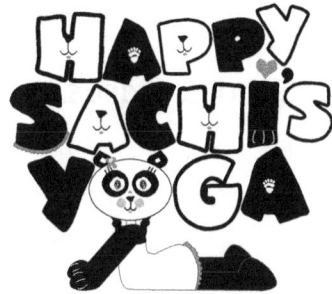

Fun Workbook 1

Sandra Clares
2013

HAPPY SACHI'S YOGA

Fun Workbook 1

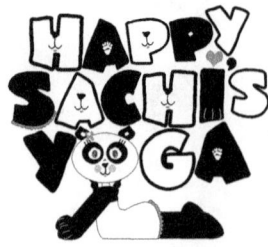

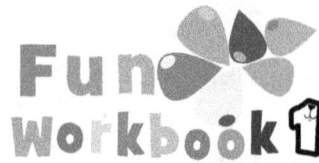

Sandra Clares
2013

HSY - Happy Sachi's Yoga

ISBN-10: 098599262X
ISBN-13: 978-0-9859926-2-0

www.happysachi.com

Printed in the United States of America

Fun Workbook 1

Imagine, color, paint, draw, illuminate, practice yoga and have lots of fun!

¡Imagina, colorea, pinta, dibuja, ilumina, practica yoga y diviértete!

HAPPY's

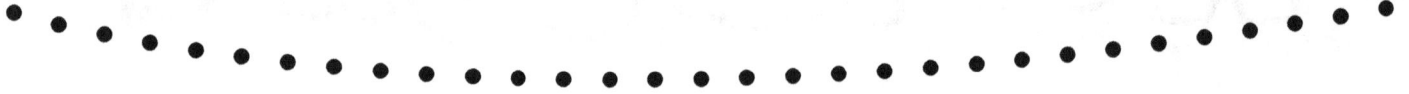

Fun Workbook 1

red - rojo

orange - naranja

Yellow - amarillo

green - verde

blue - azul

violet - violeta

Pink - rosa

purple - morado

fuchsia - fucsia

aqua - aguamarina

grey - gris

White - blanco

black - negro

brown - café

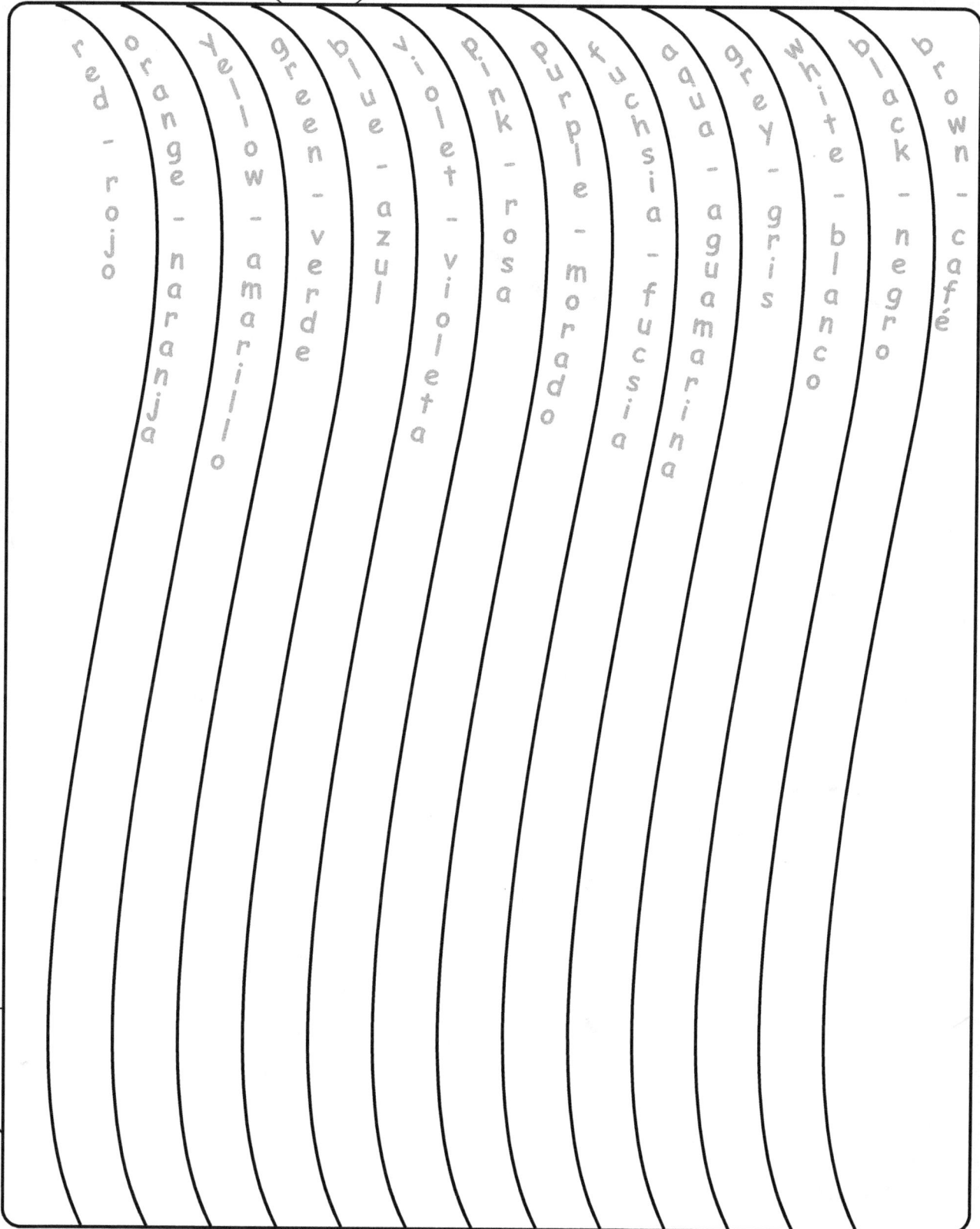

Rainbow - Arcoíris

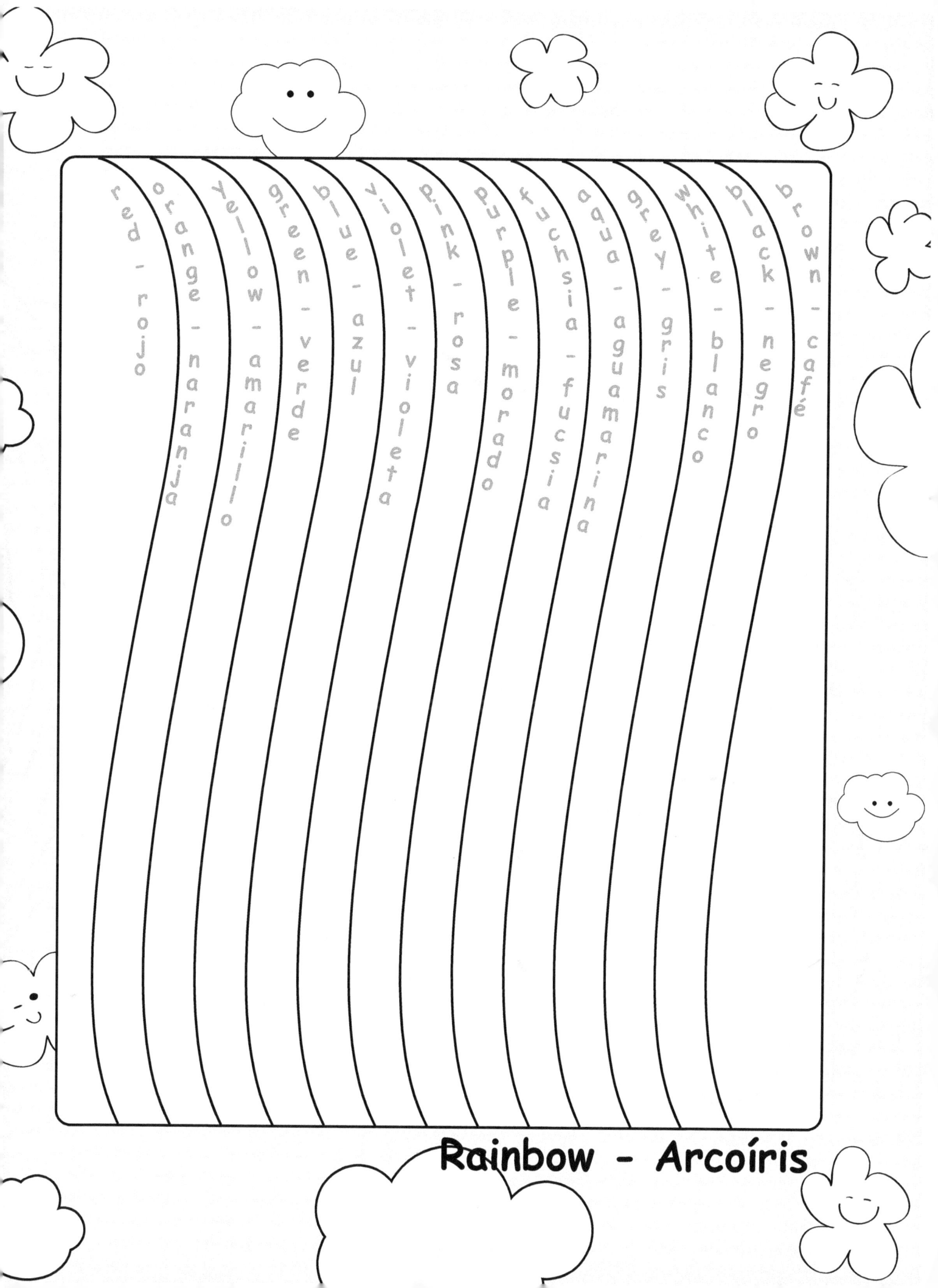

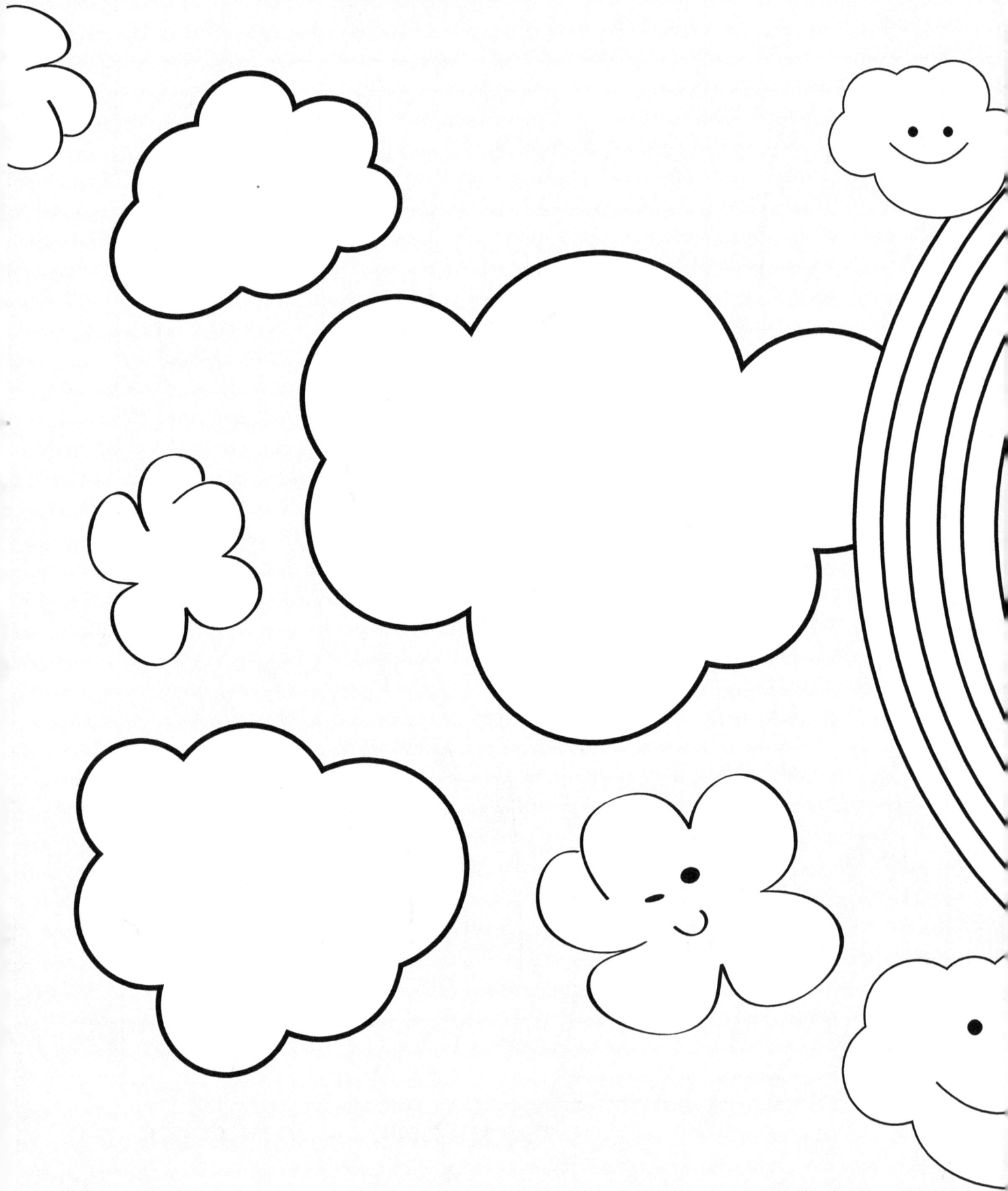

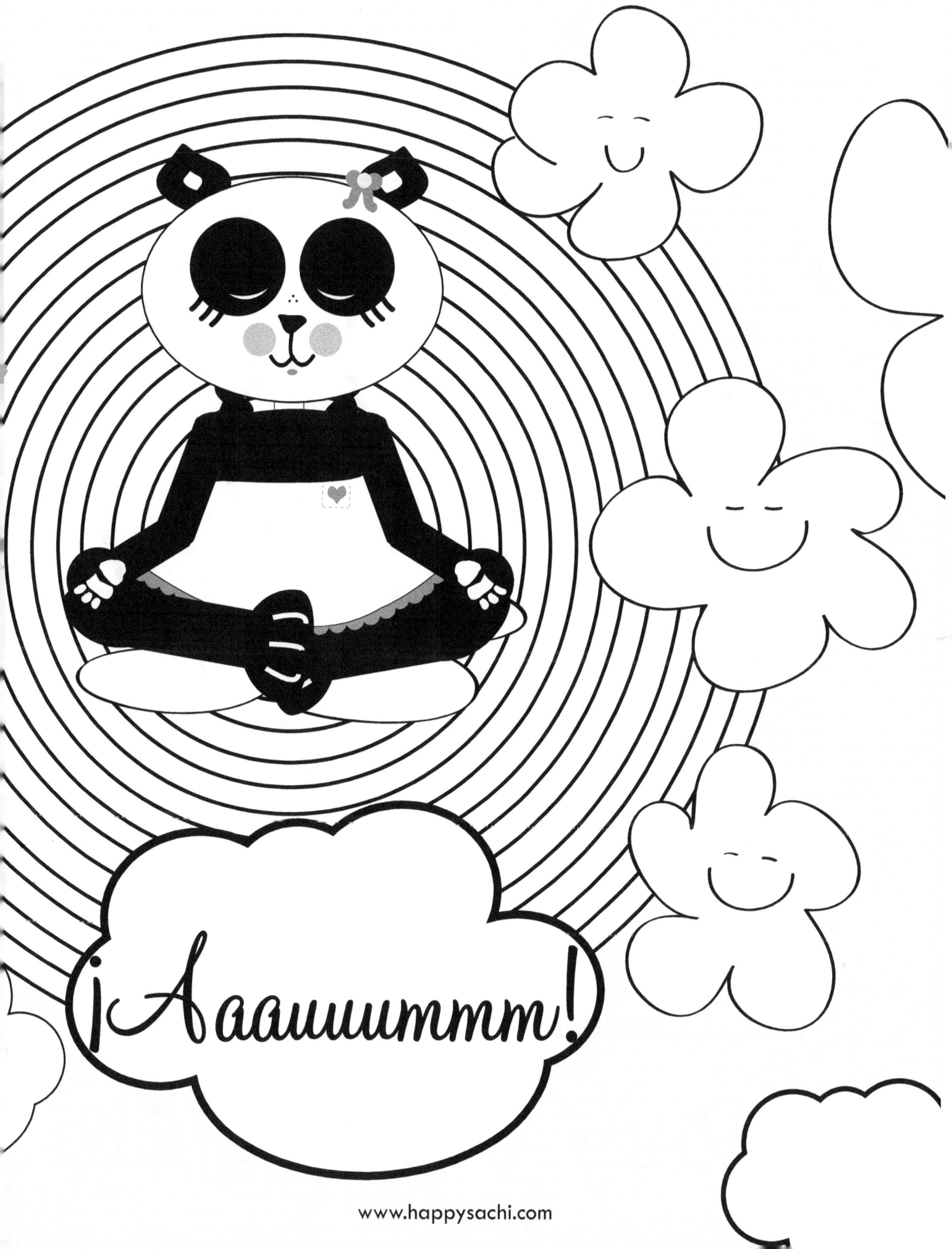

¡Aauuummm!

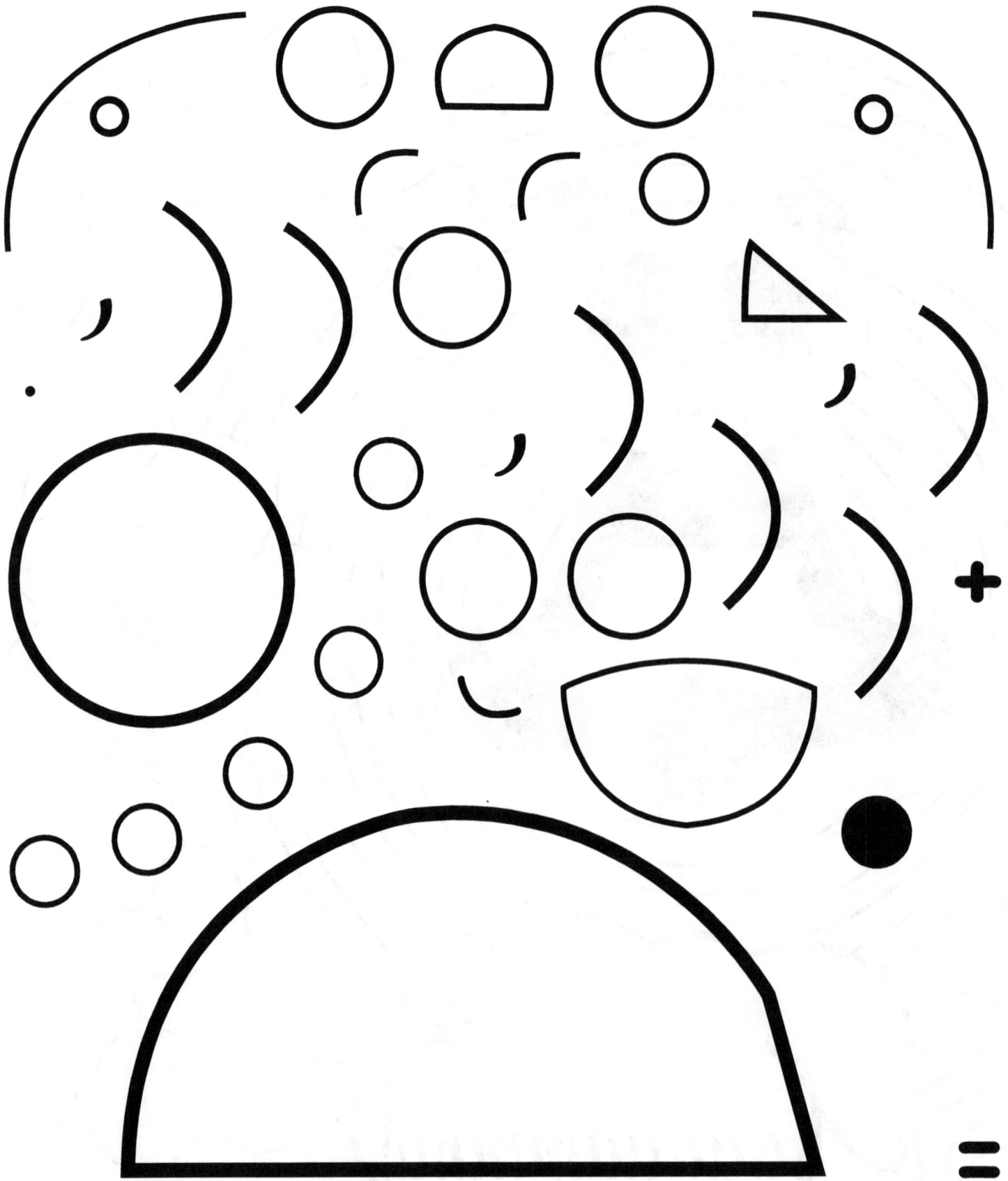

ladybug - mariquita

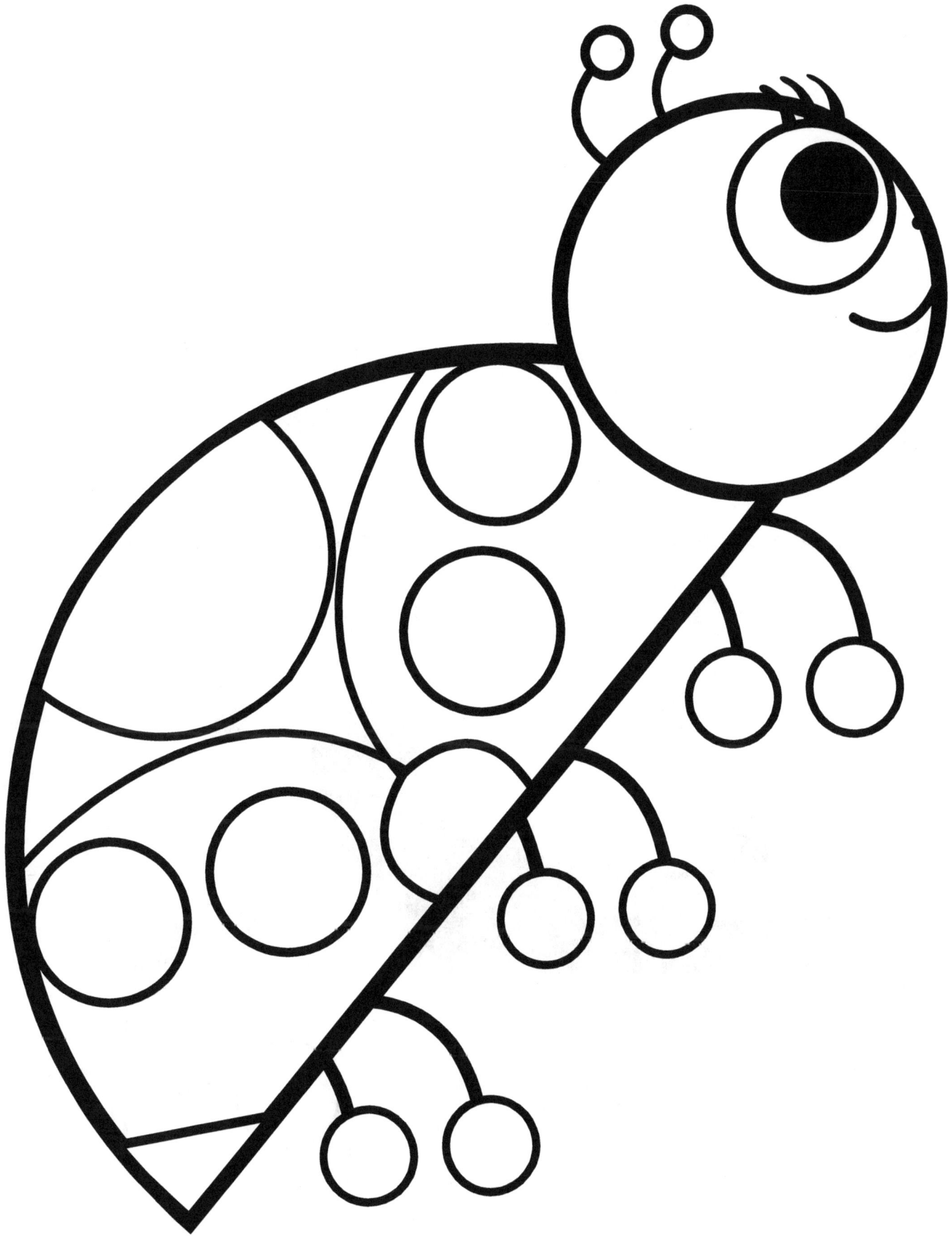

ladybug - mariquita

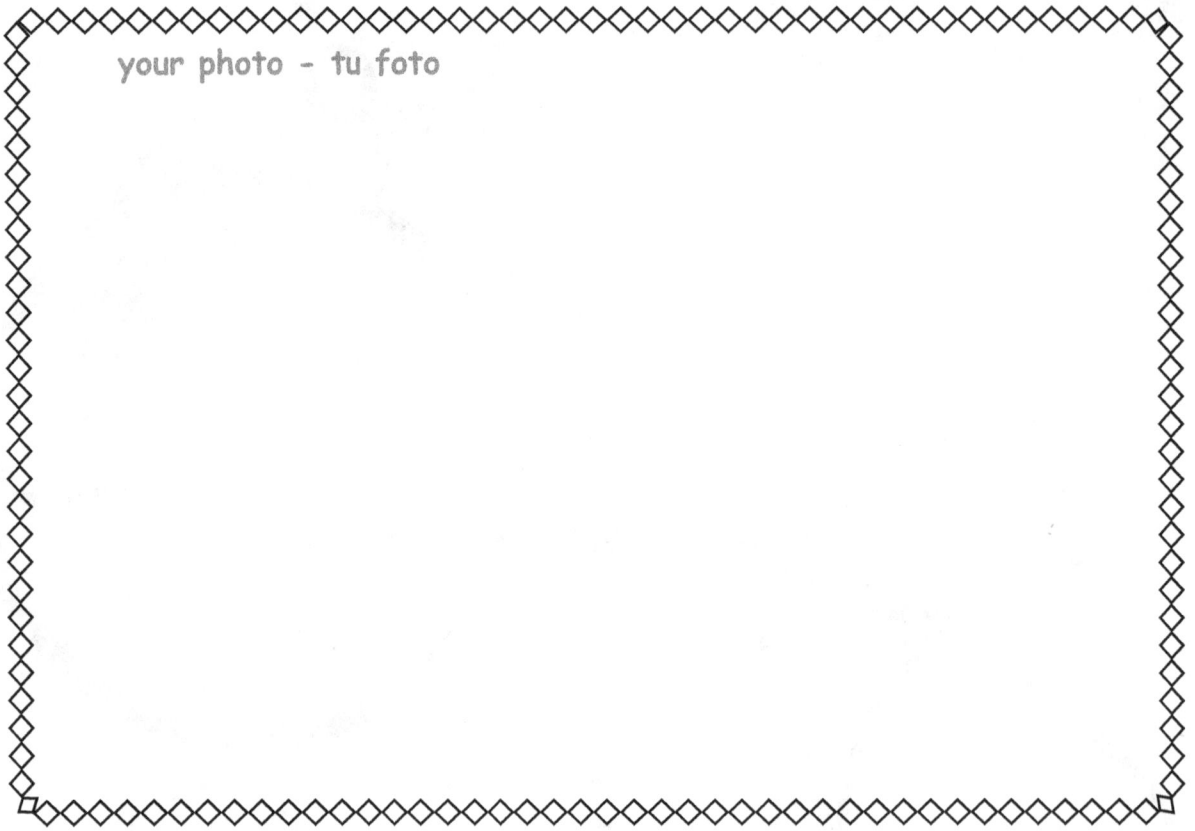

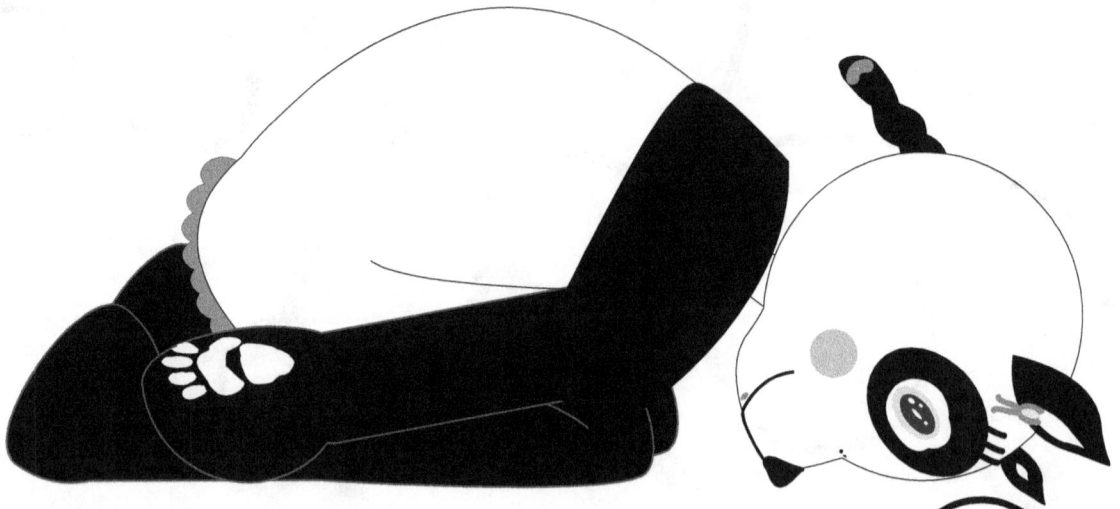

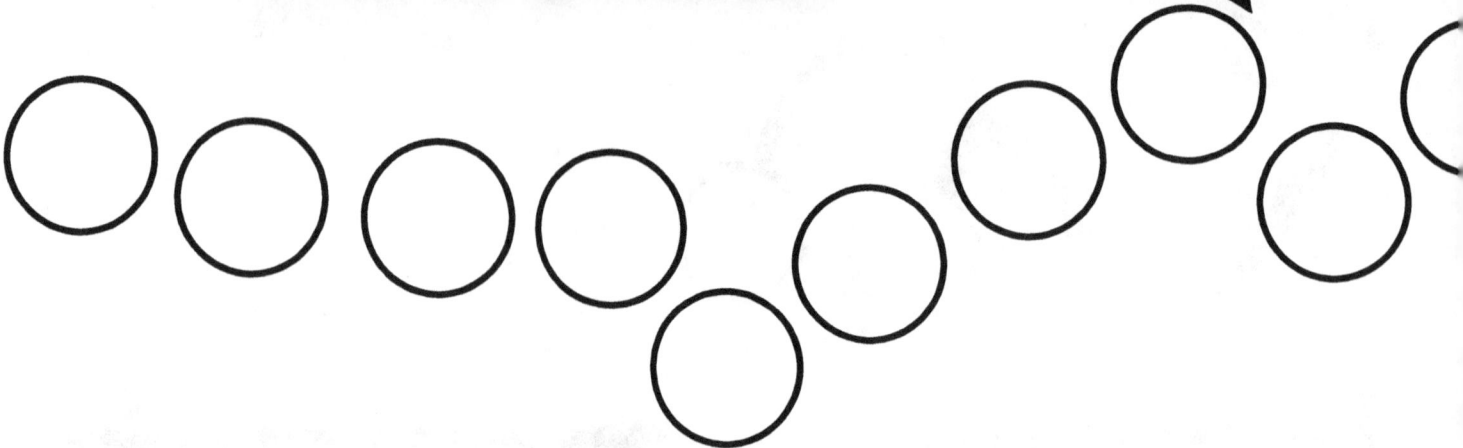

ladybug - mariquita

Happy Sachi's Yoga

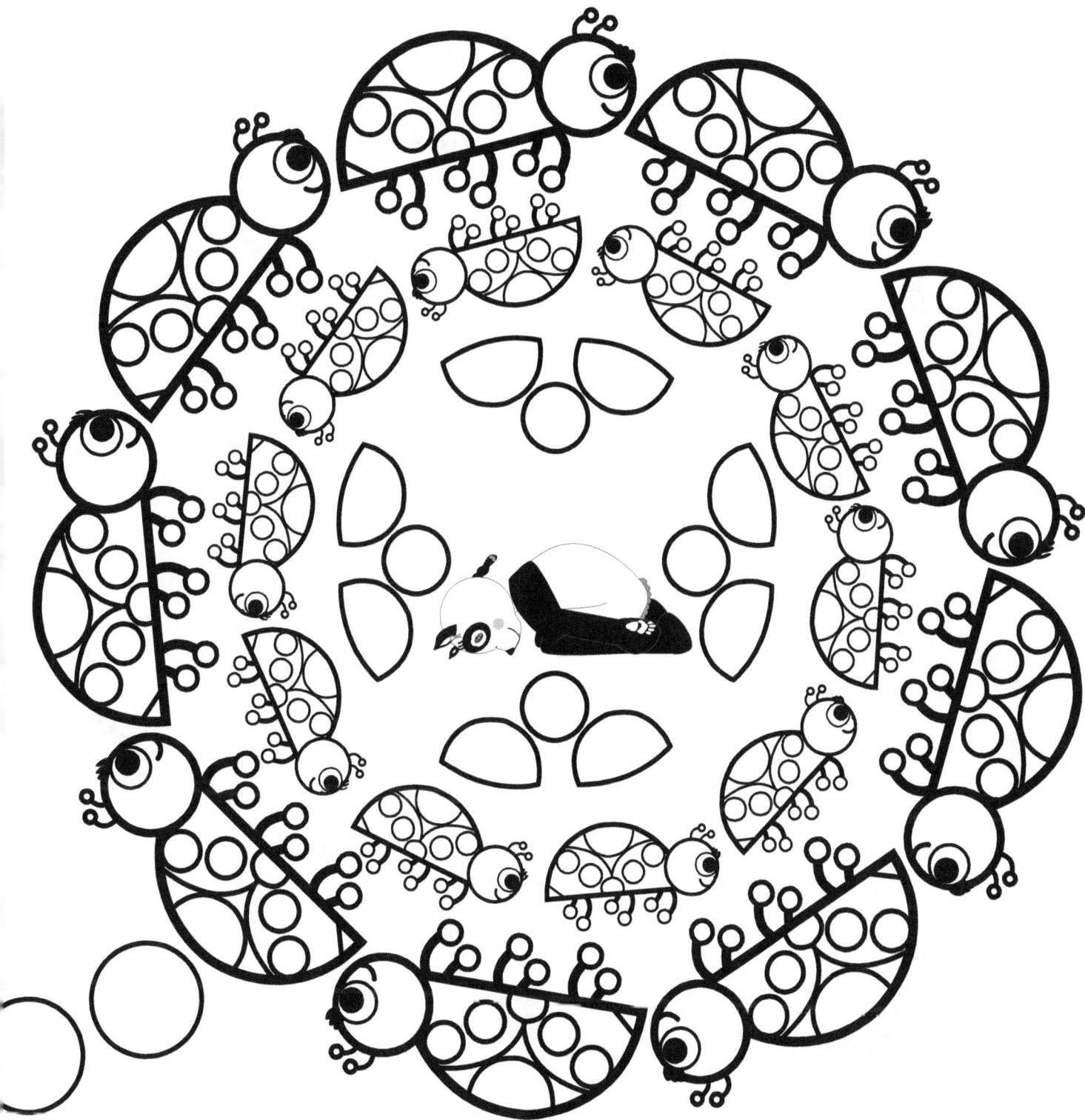

ladybug - mariquita

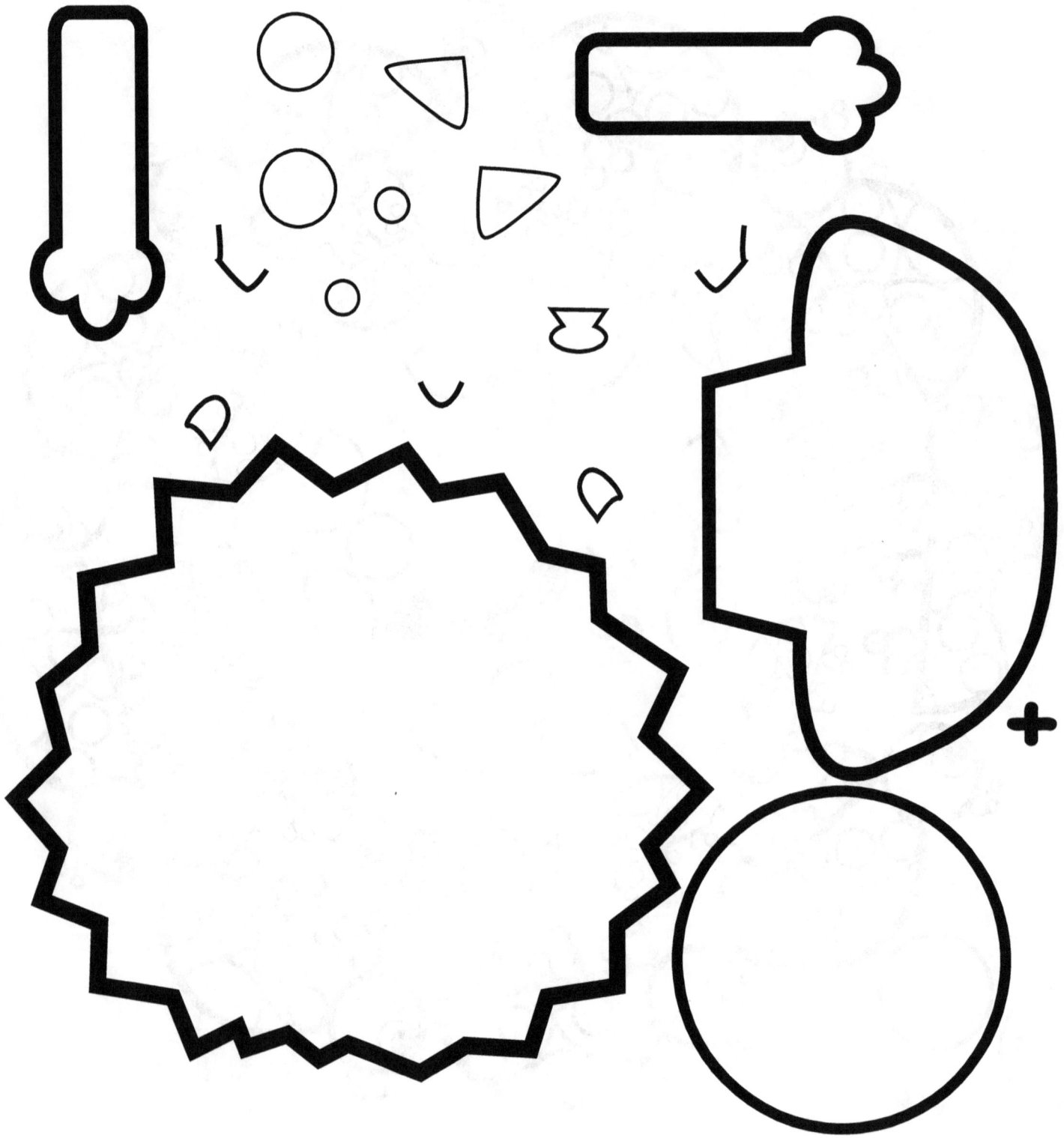

lion - león

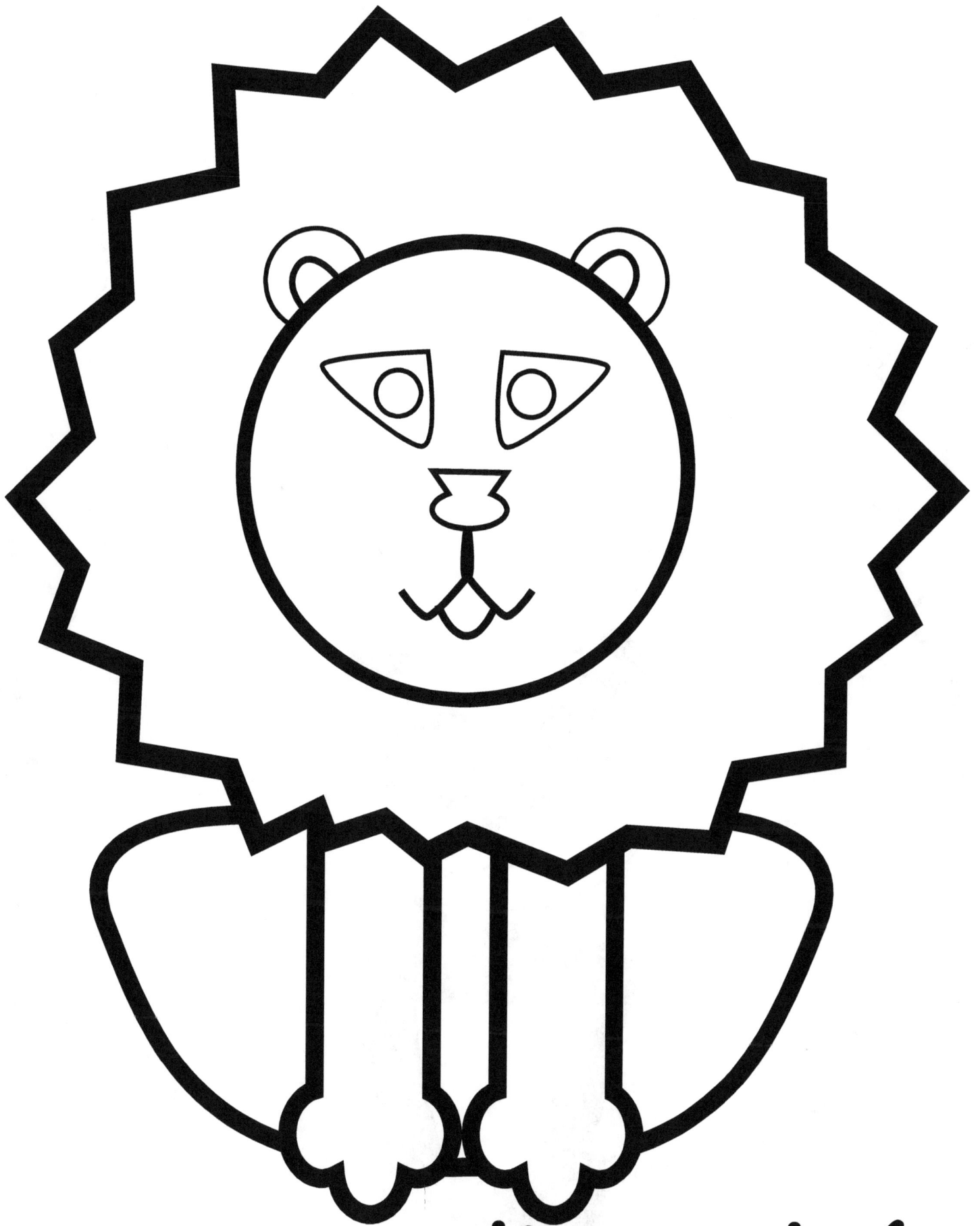

lion - león

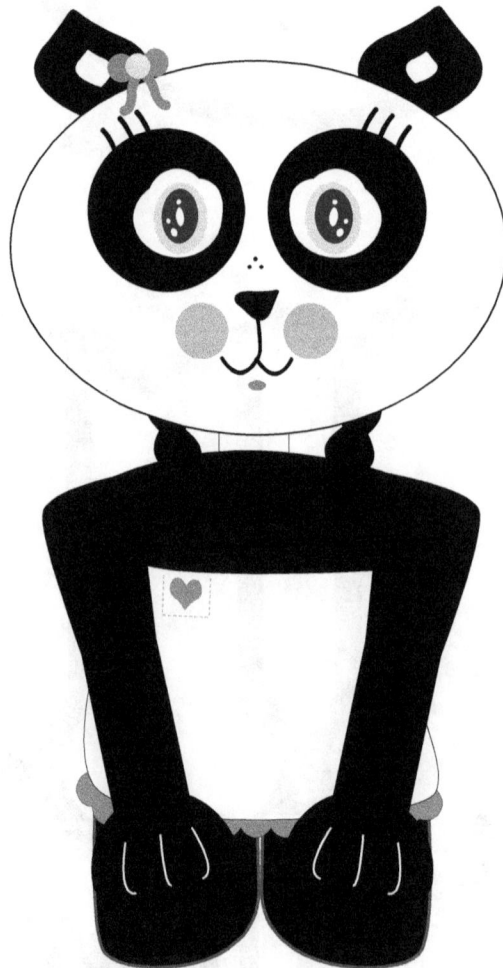

lion - león

Happy Sachi's Yoga

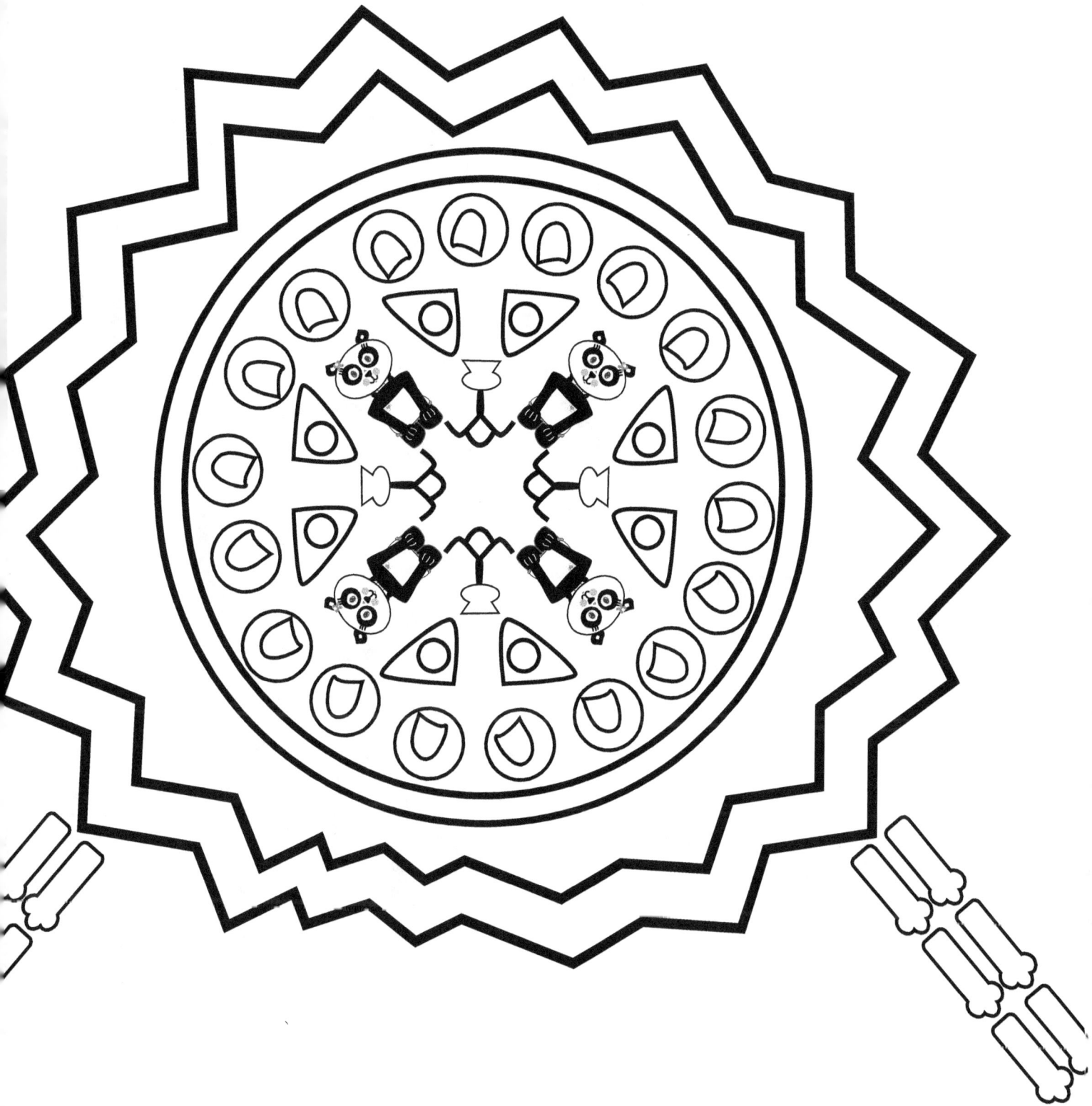

lion - león

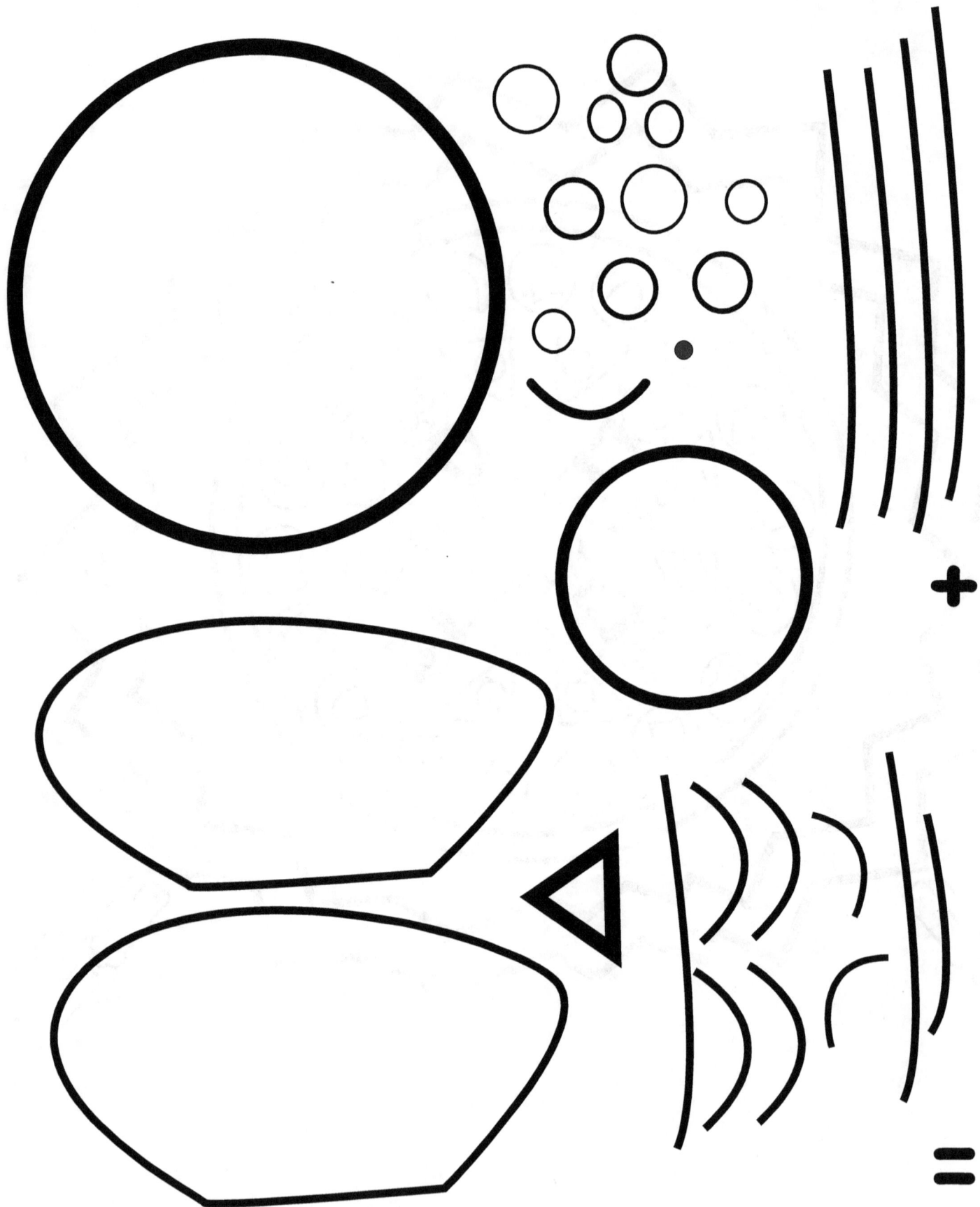

bee - abeja

Happy Sachi's Yoga

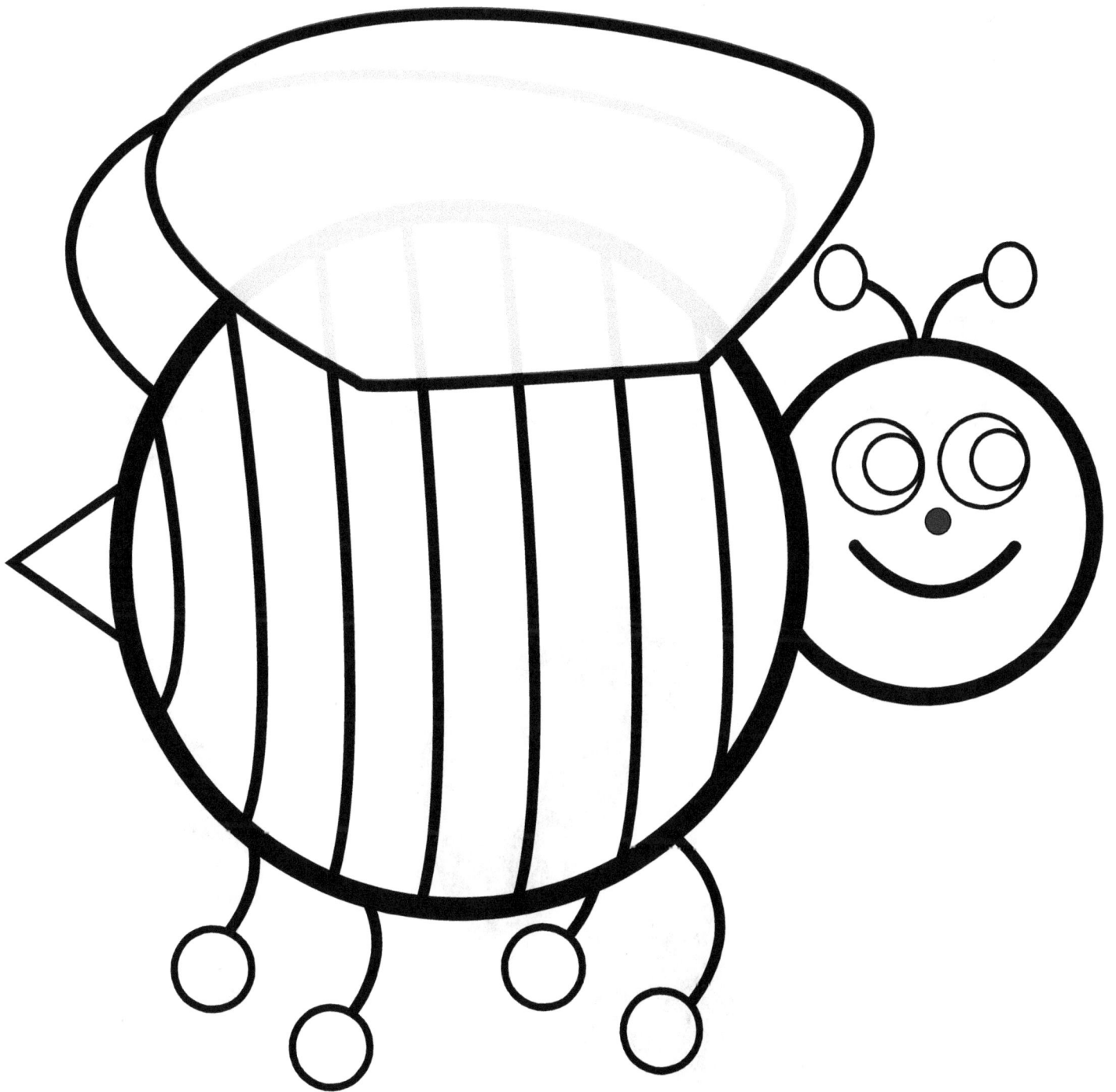

bee - abeja

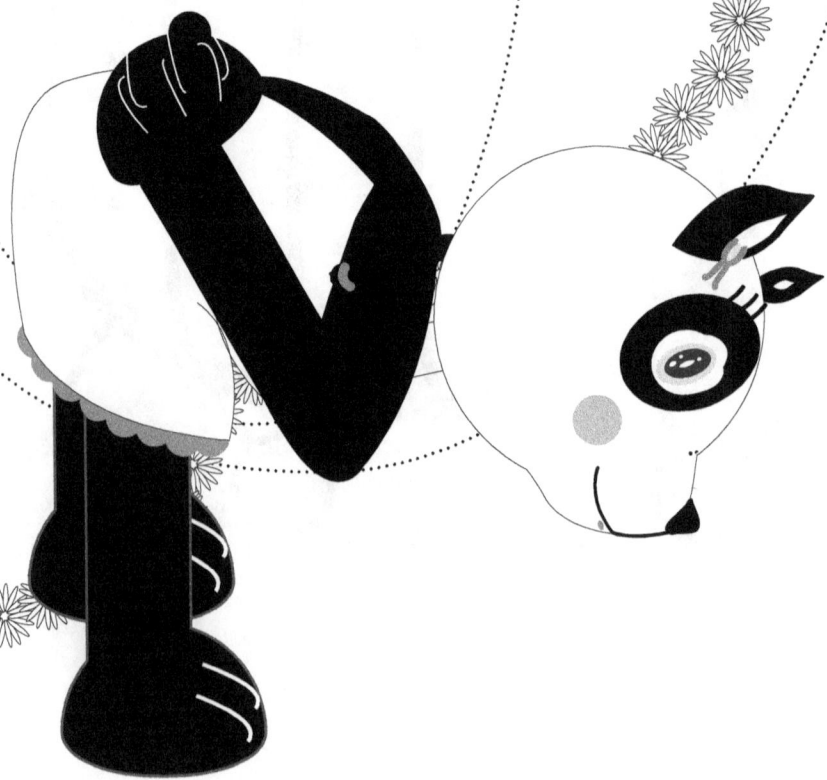

bee - abeja

Happy Sachi's Yoga

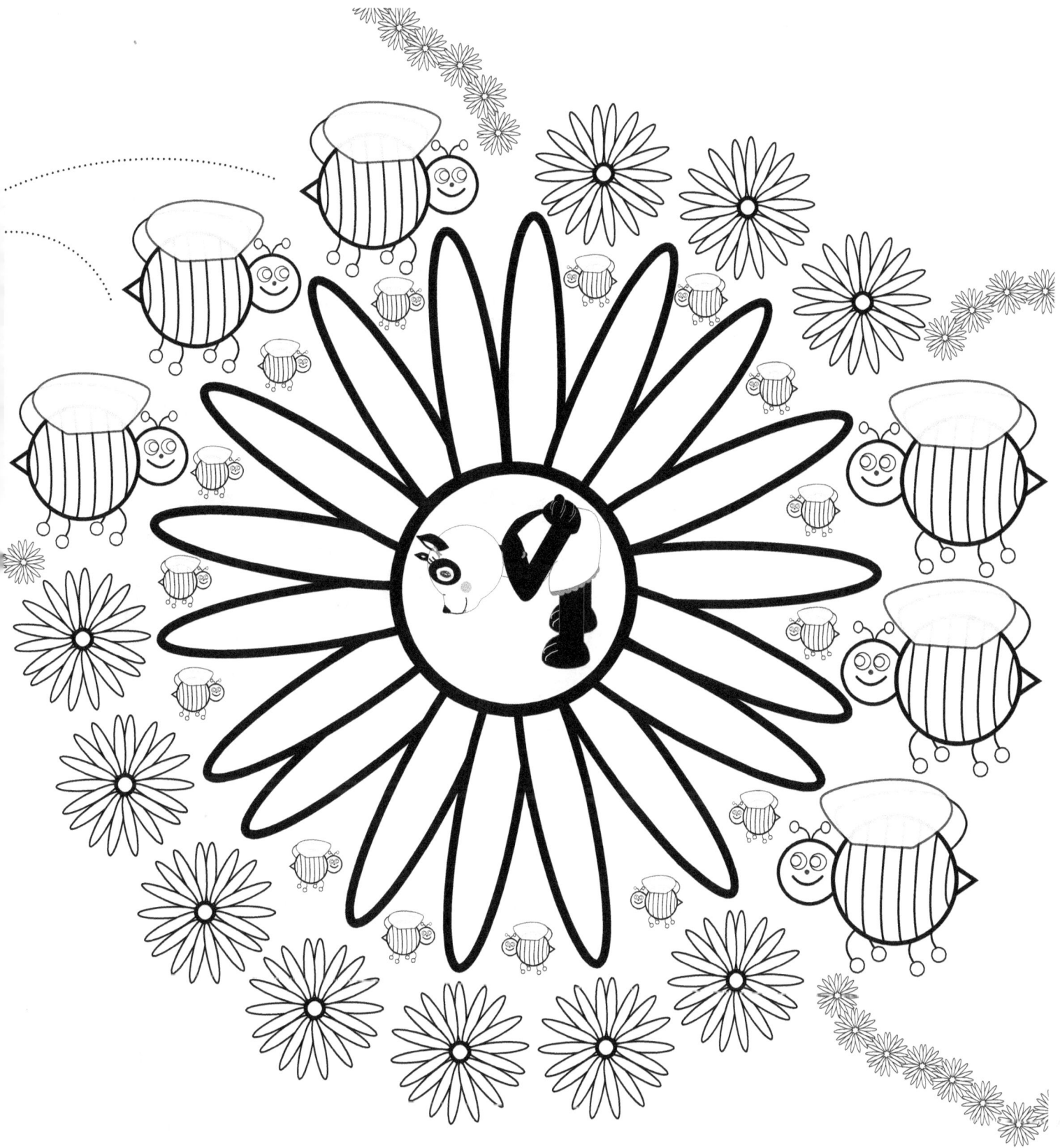

bee - abeja

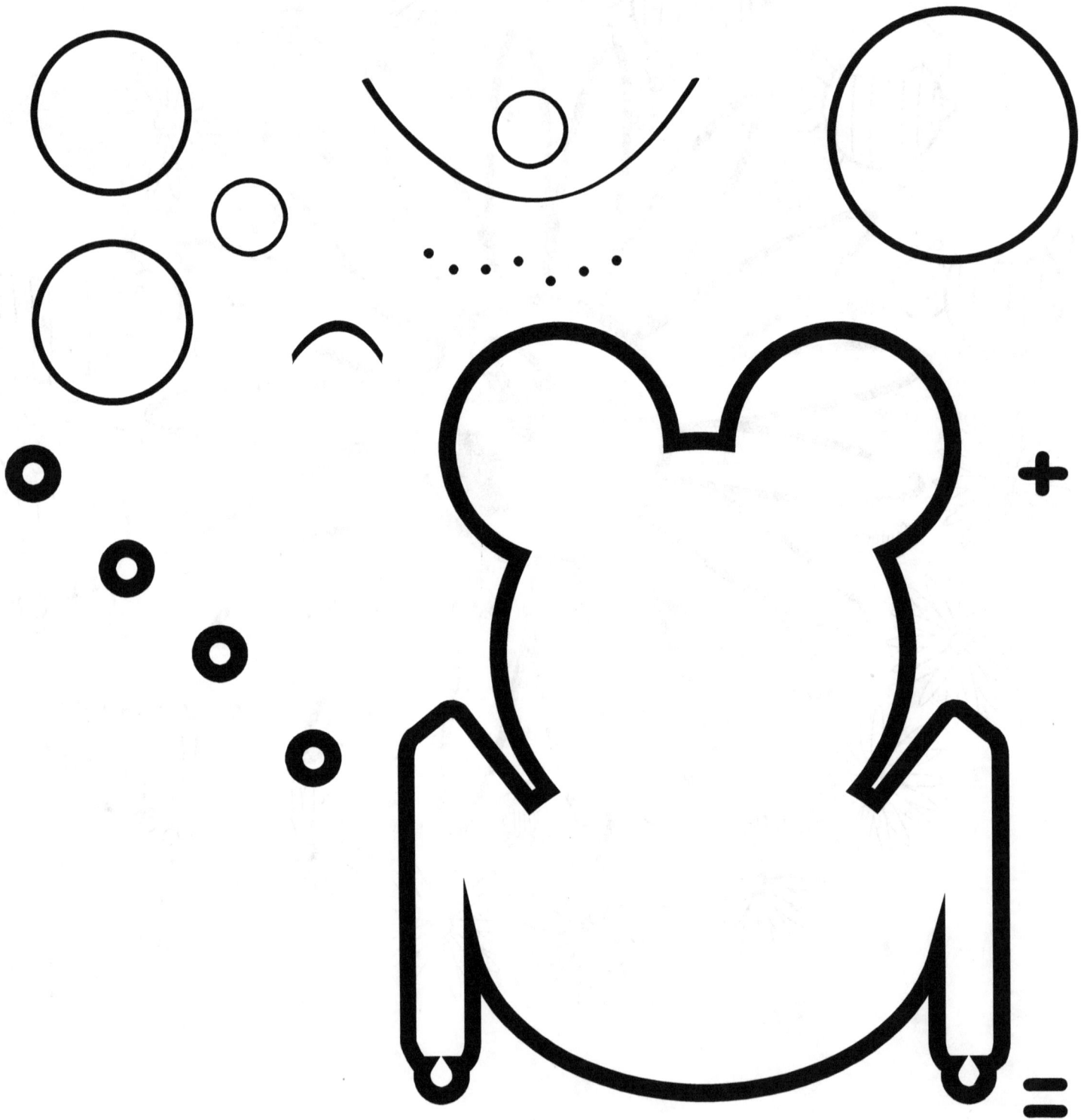

frog - rana

Happy Sachi's Yoga

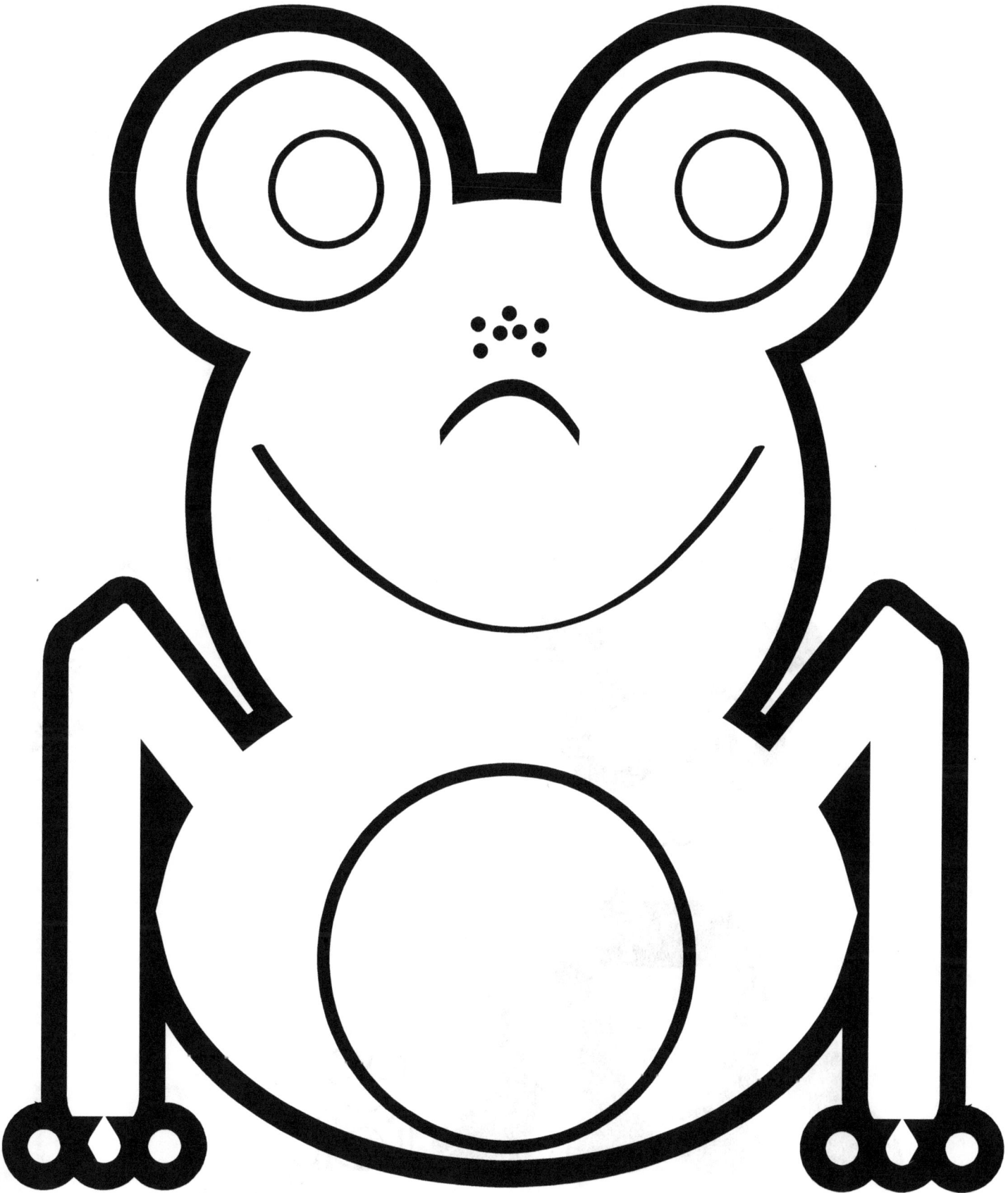

frog - rana

draw yourself - dibujate

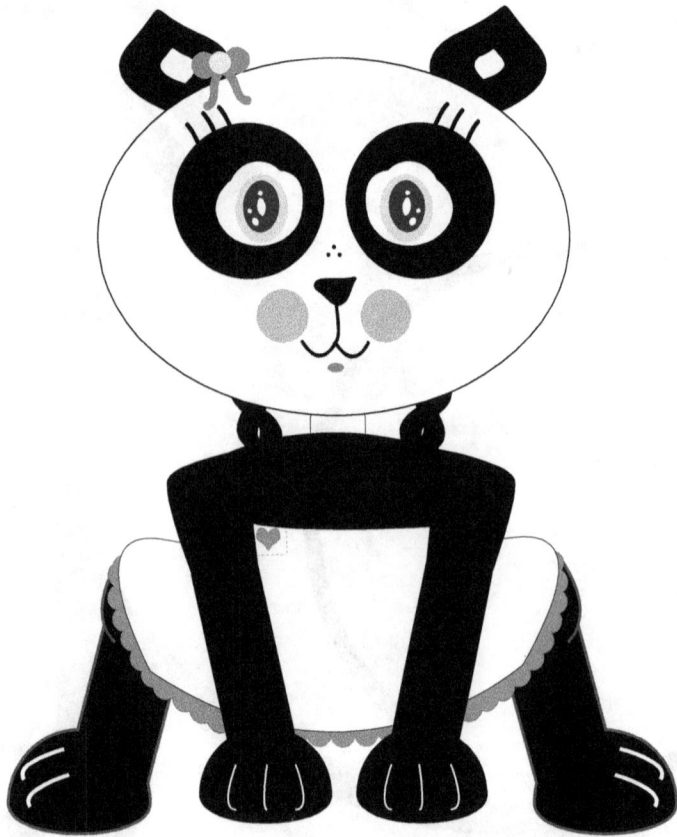

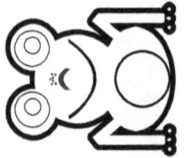

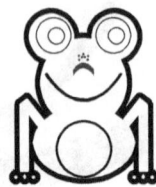

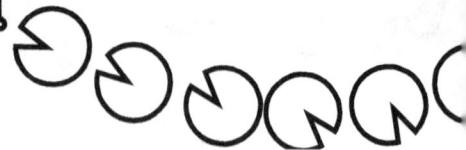

frog - rana

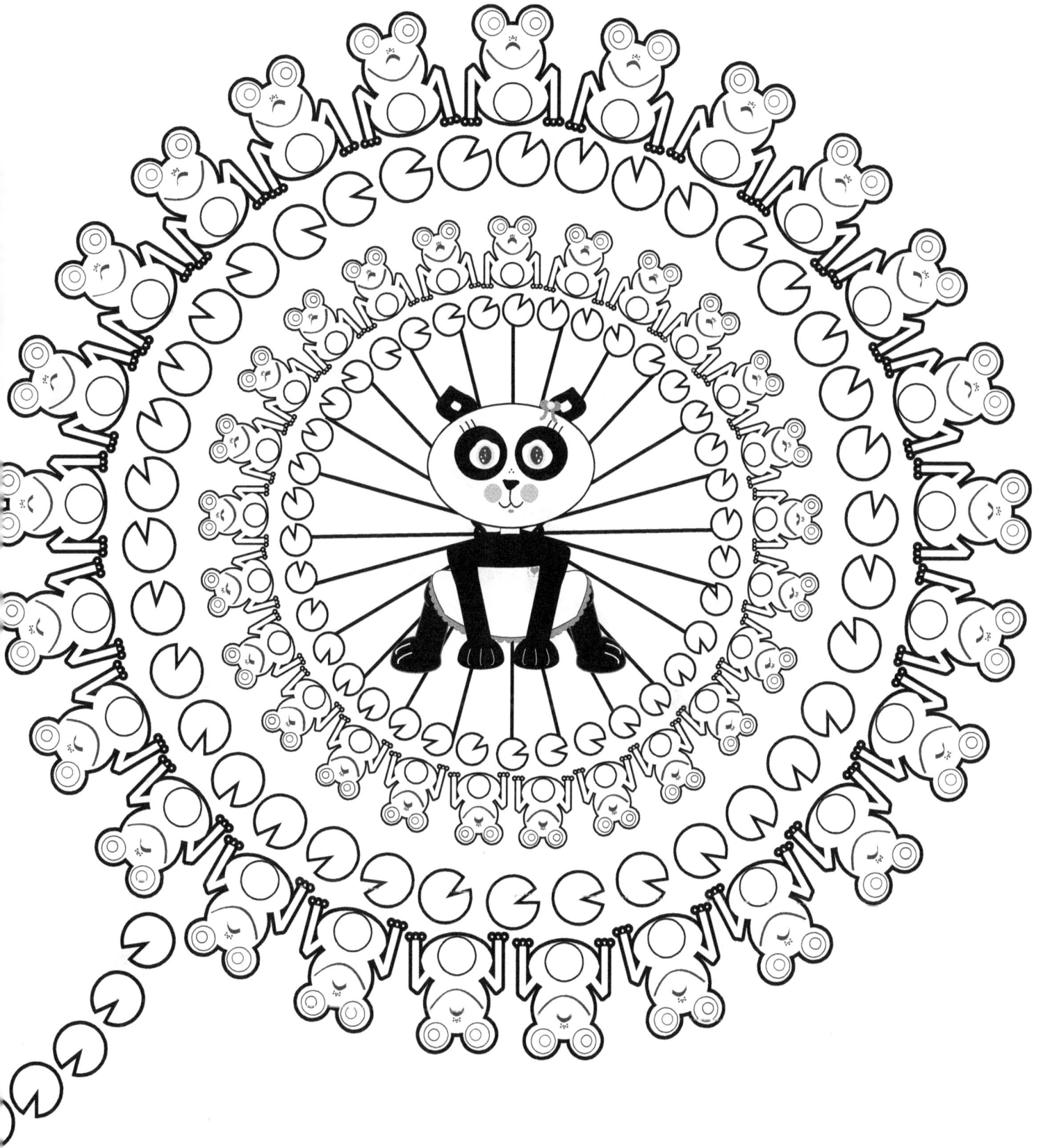

frog - rana

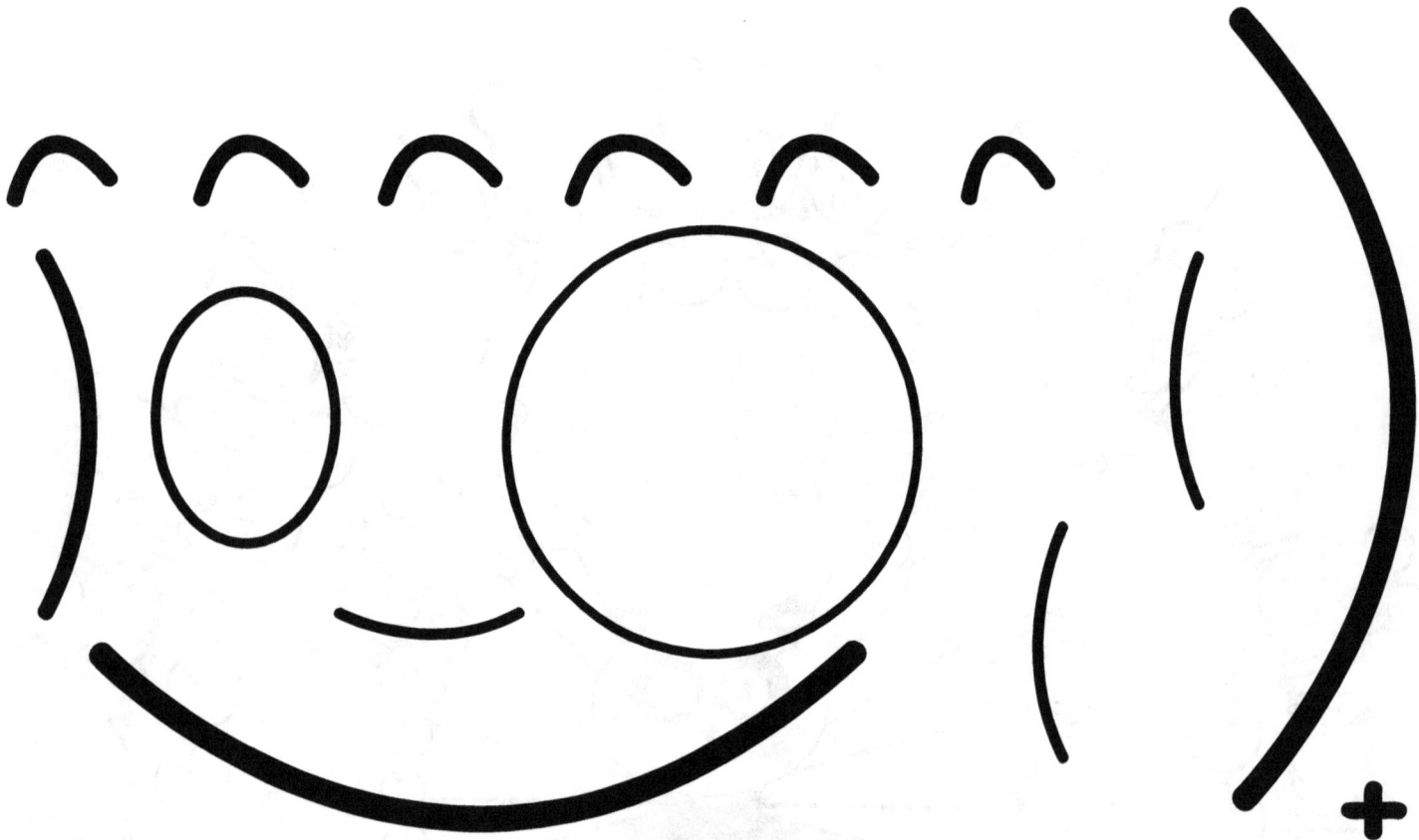

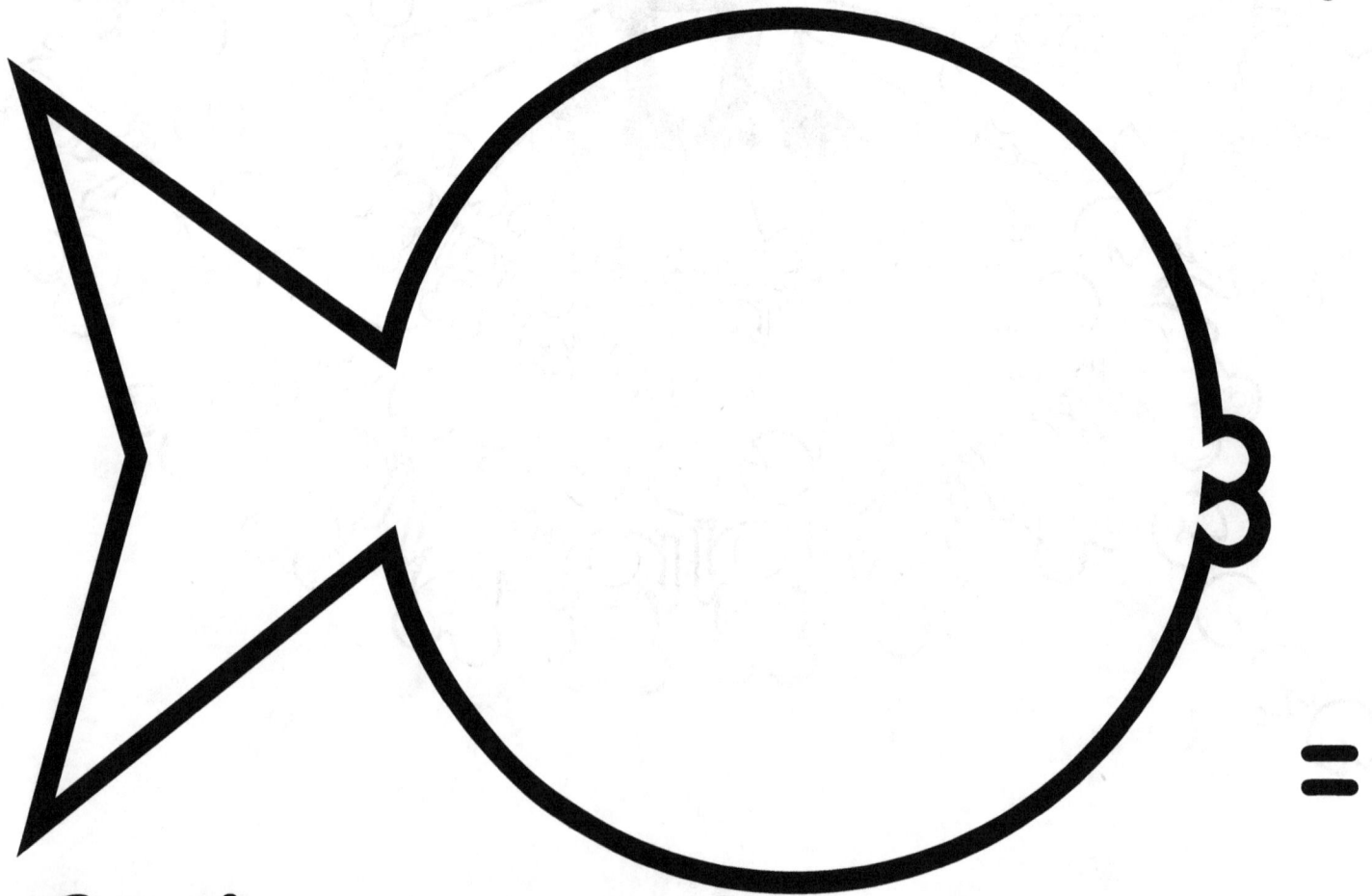

+

=

fish - pez

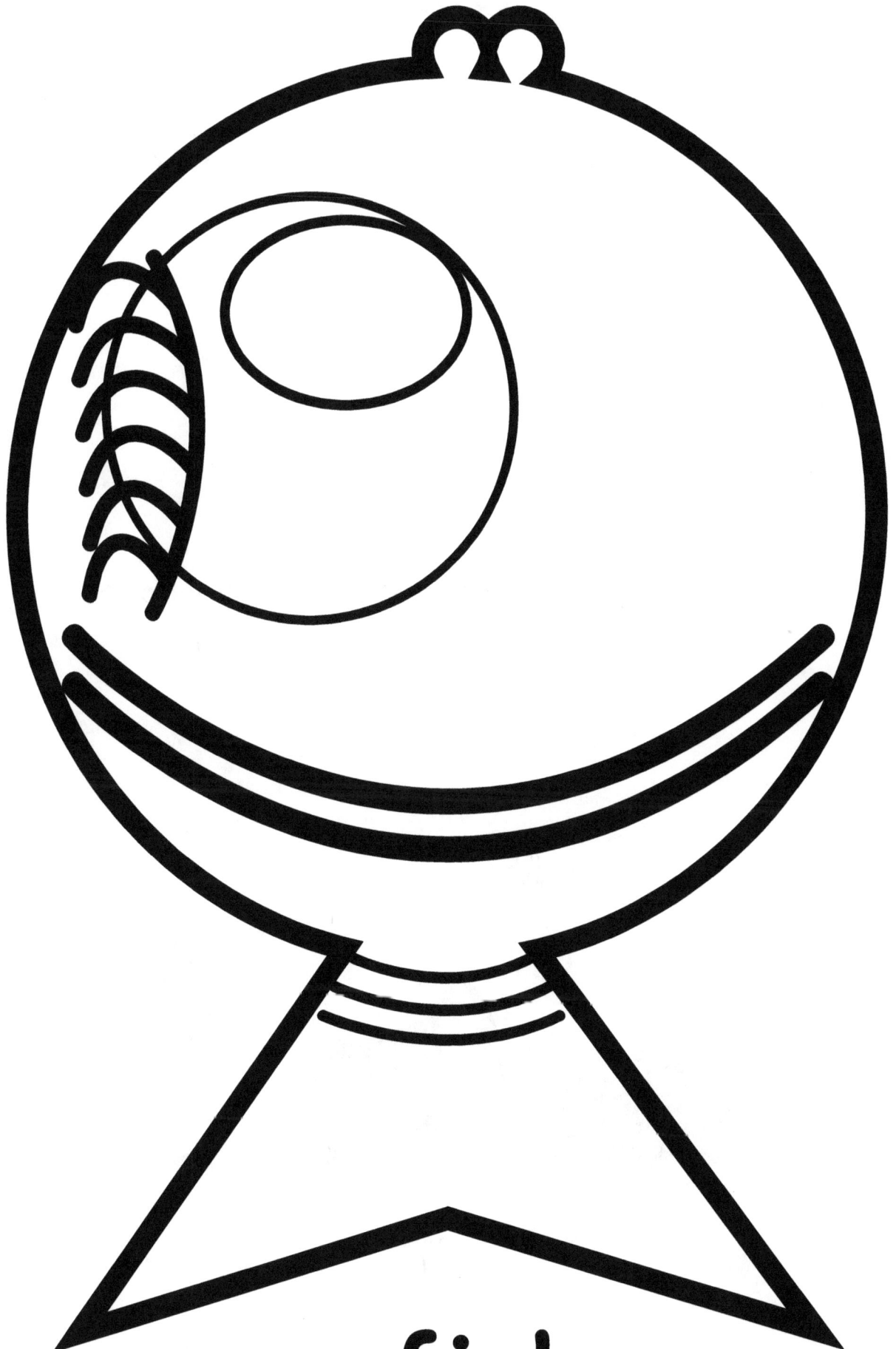

fish - pez

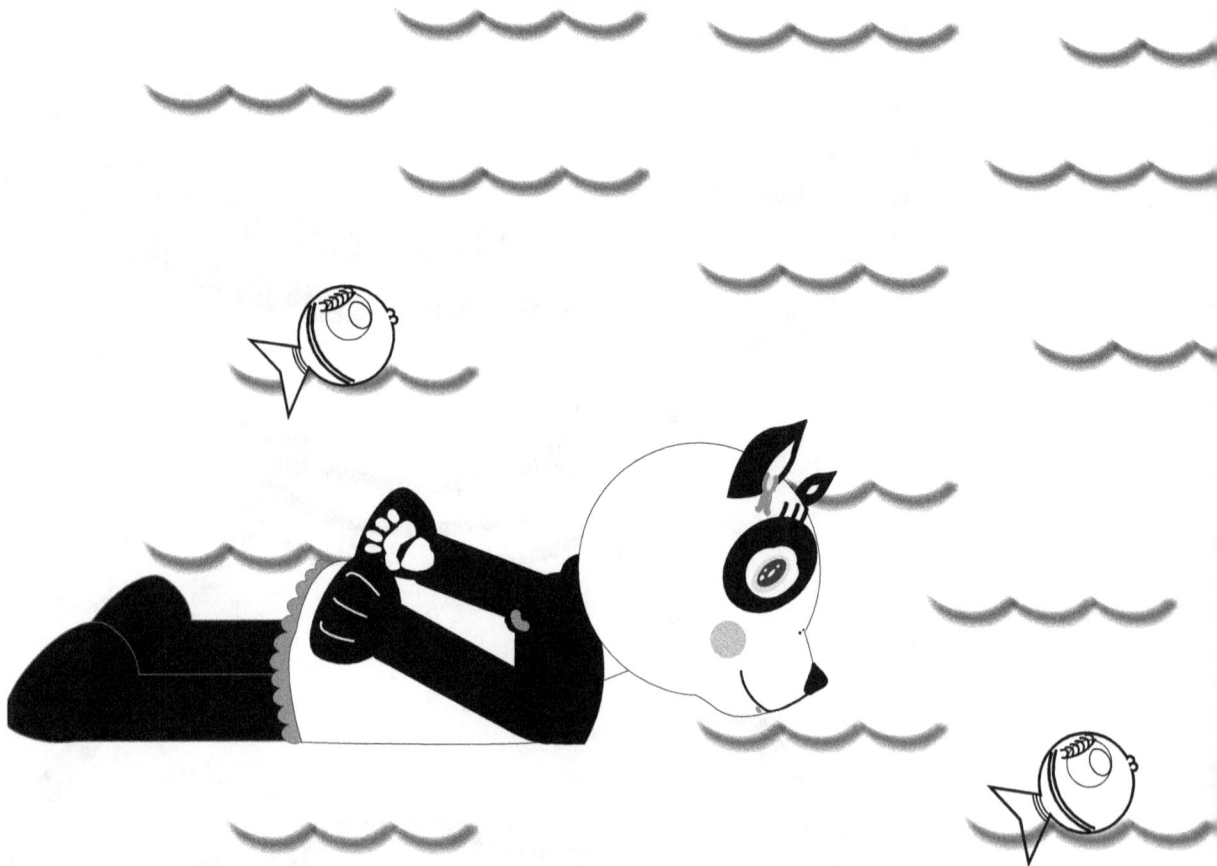

fish - pez

Happy Sachi's Yoga

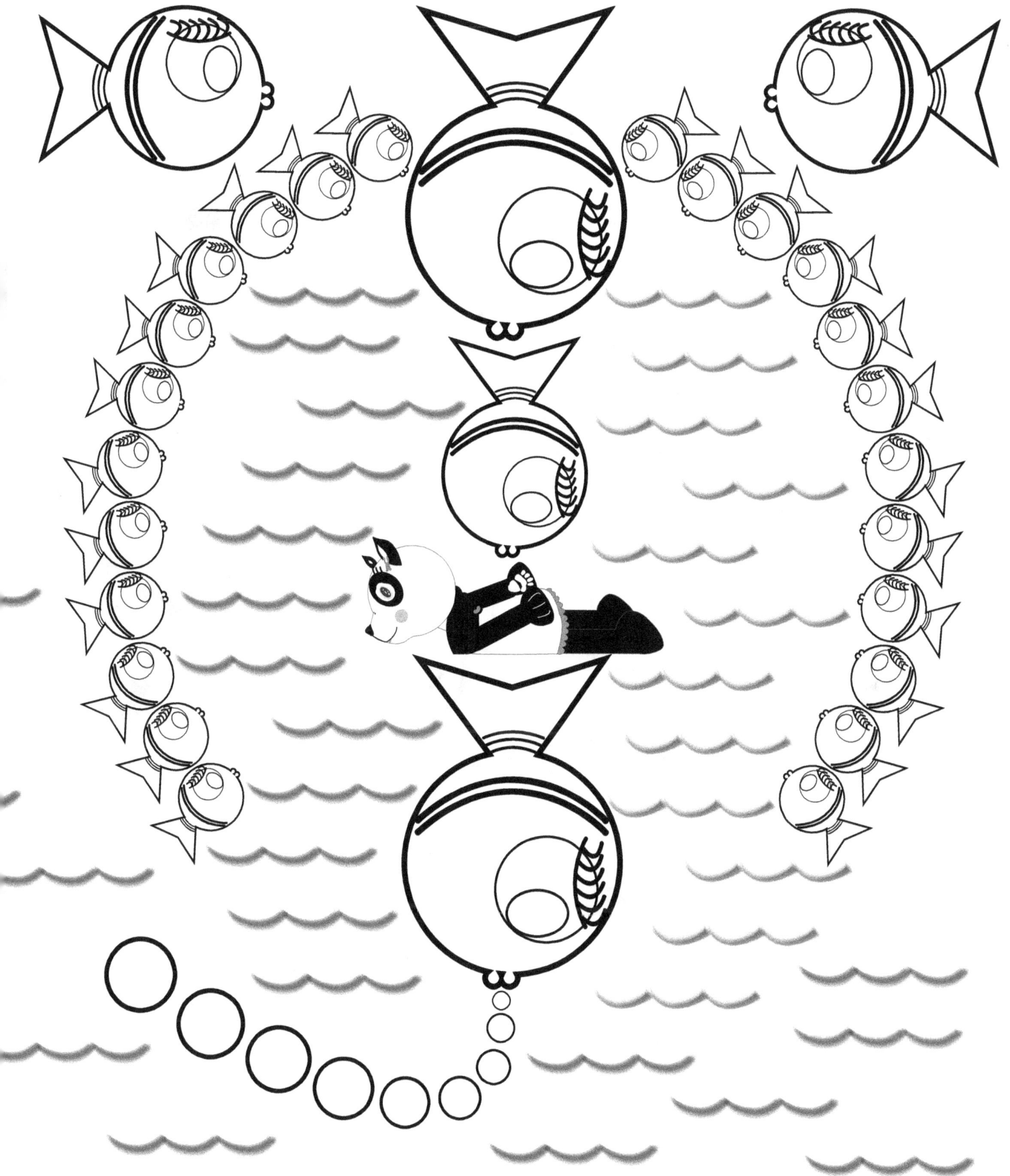

fish - pez

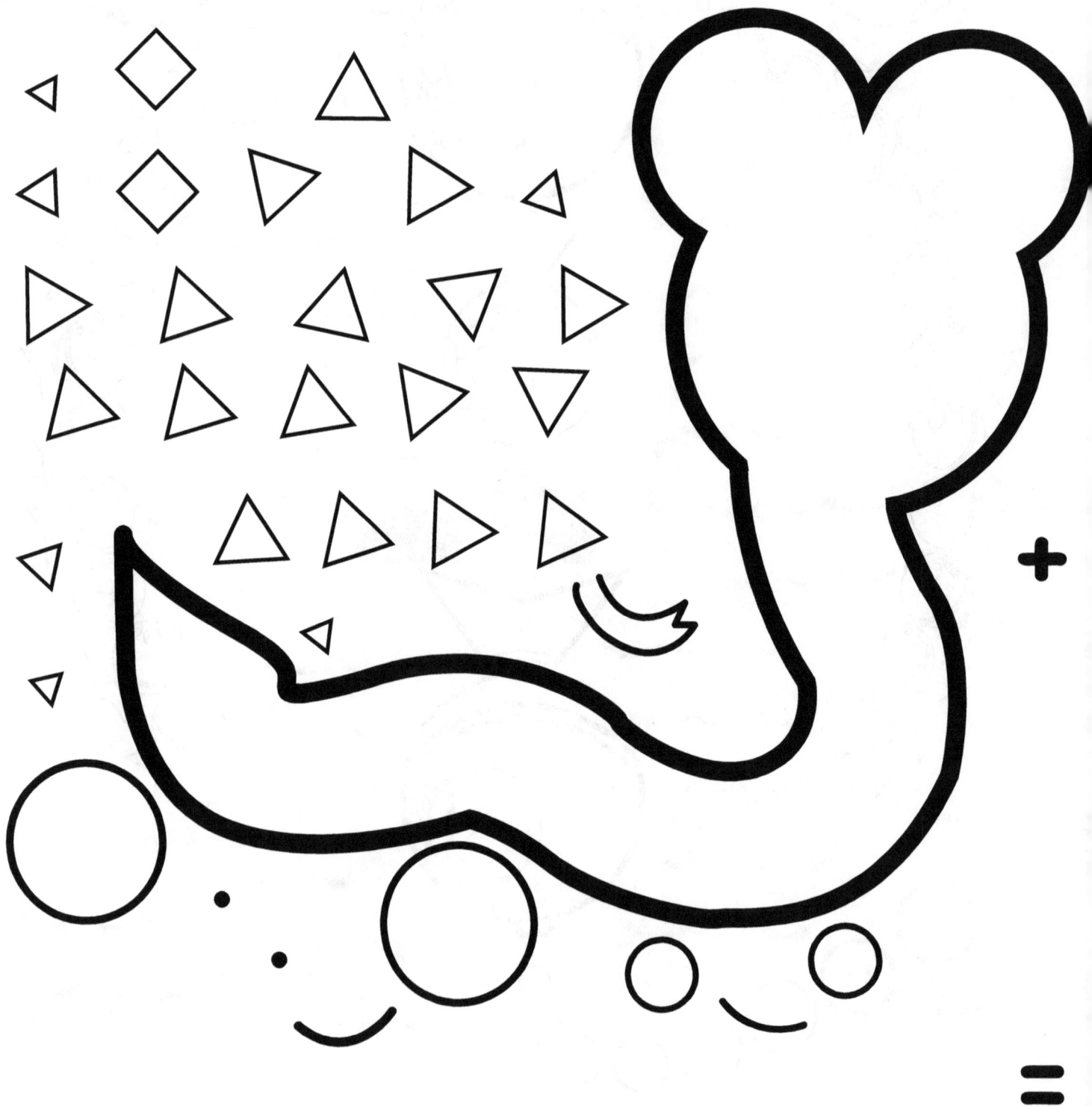

+

=

snake - víbora

Happy Sachi's Yoga

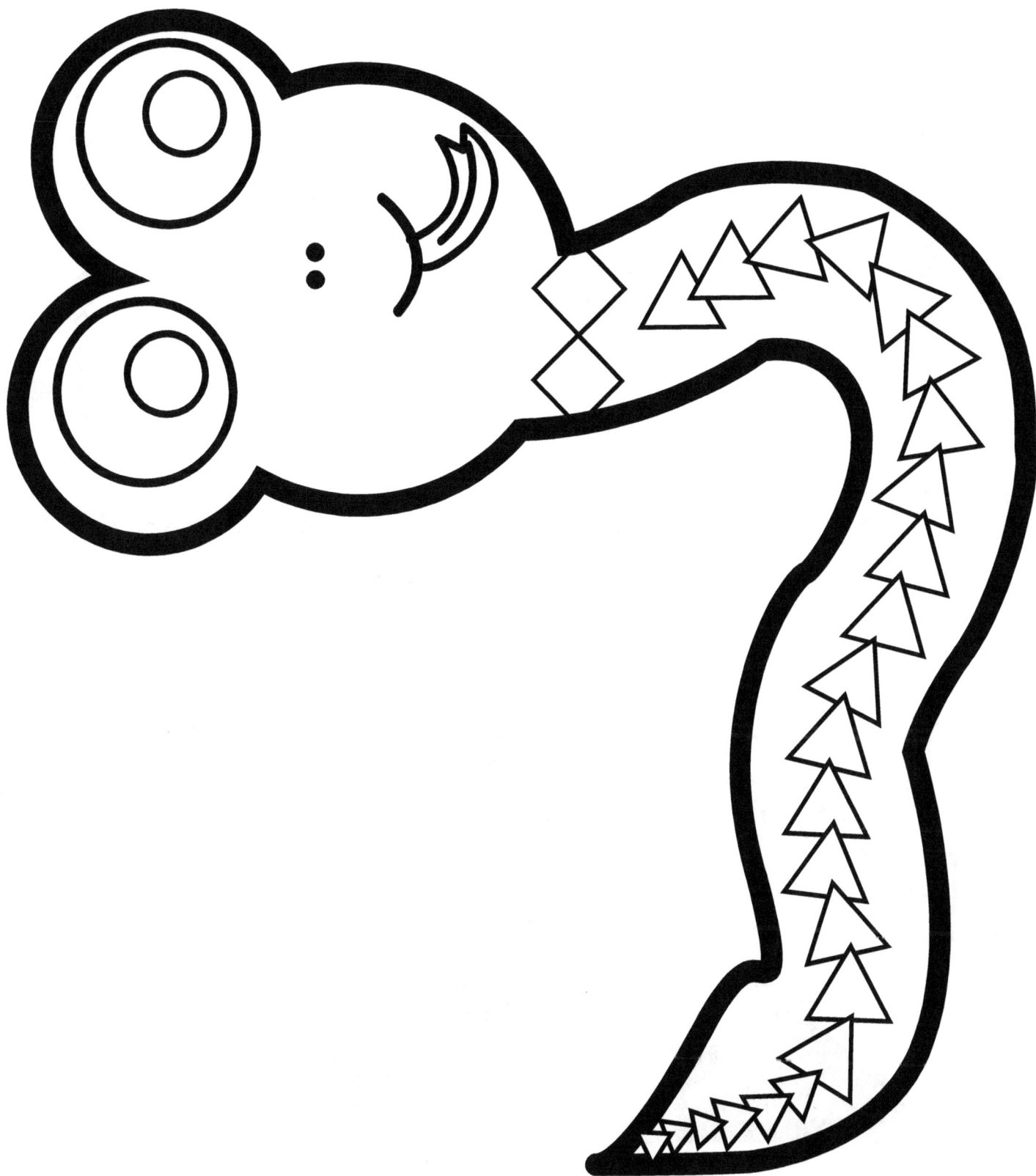

snake - víbora

draw yourself - dibujate

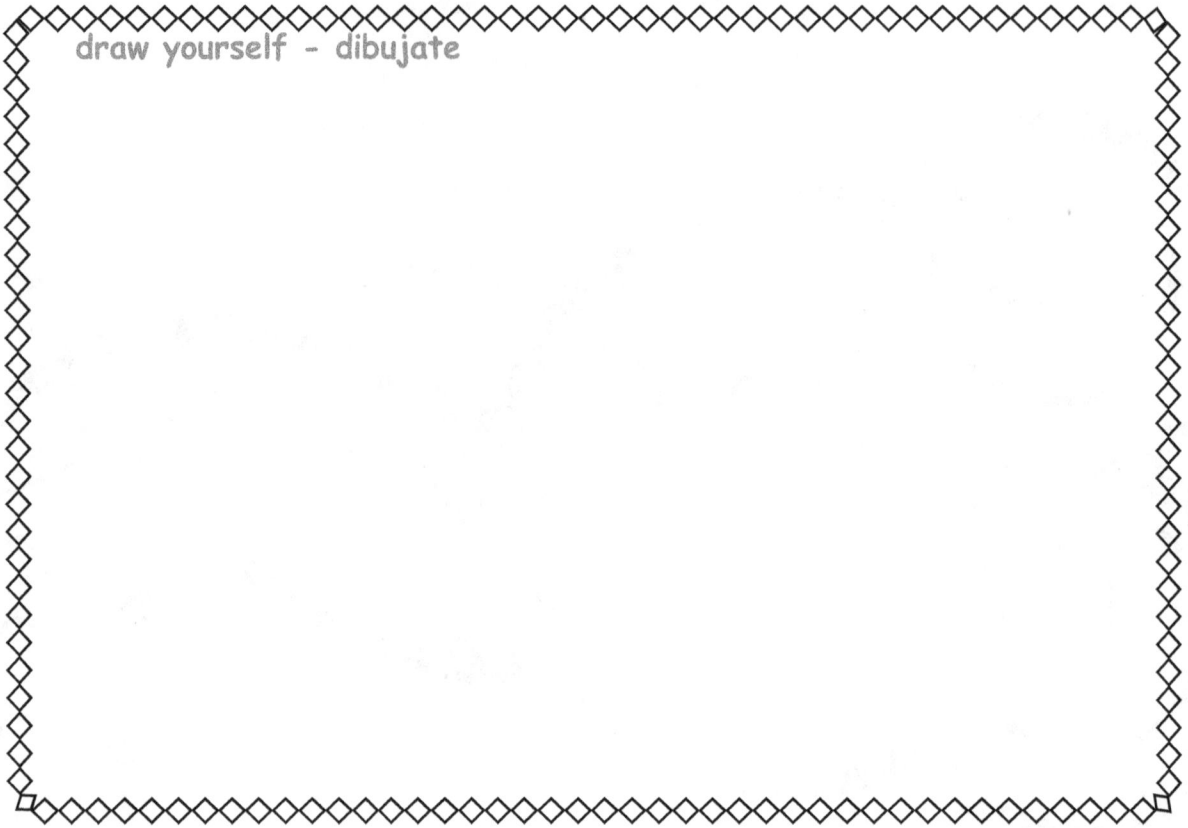

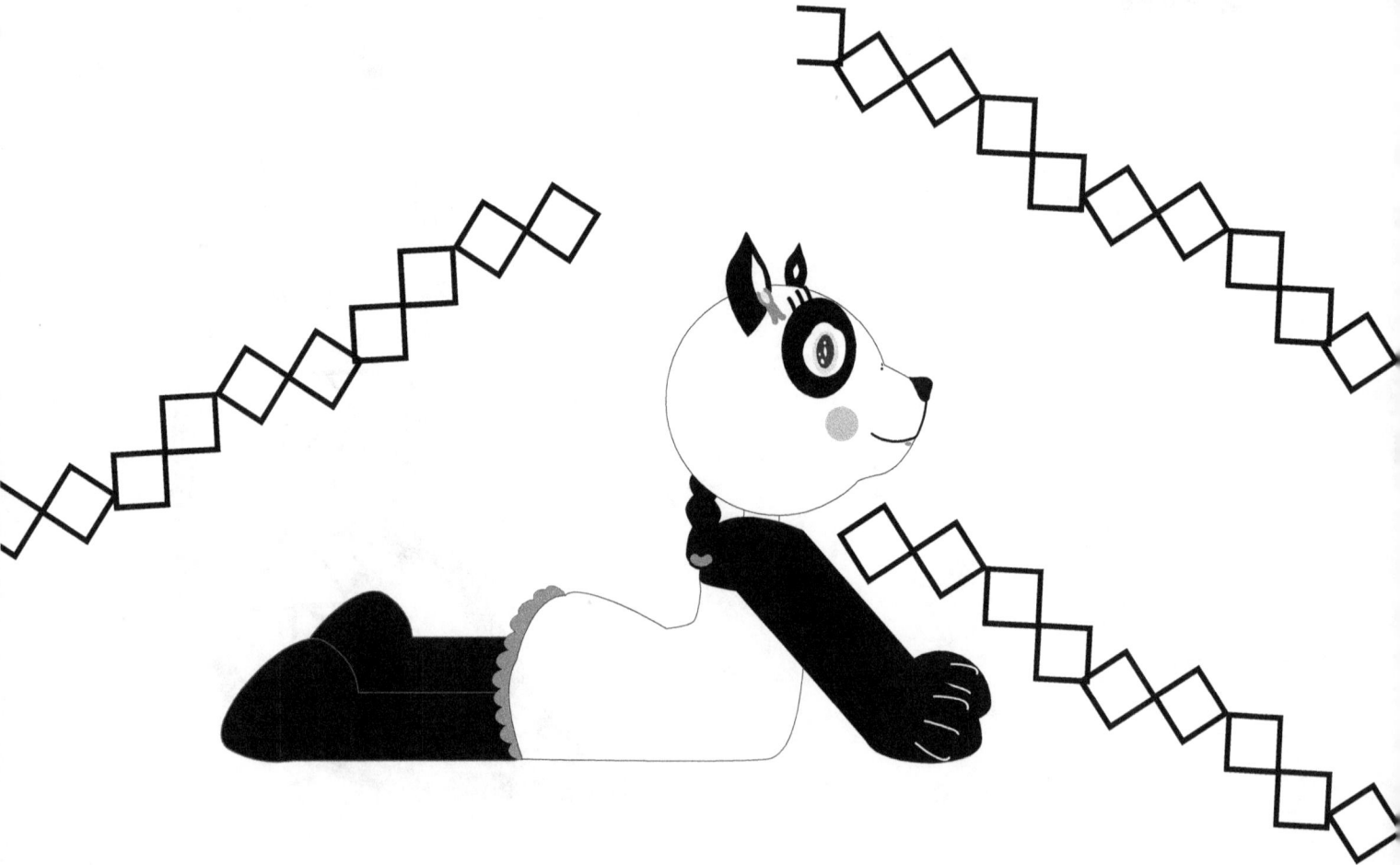

snake - víbora

Happy Sachi's Yoga

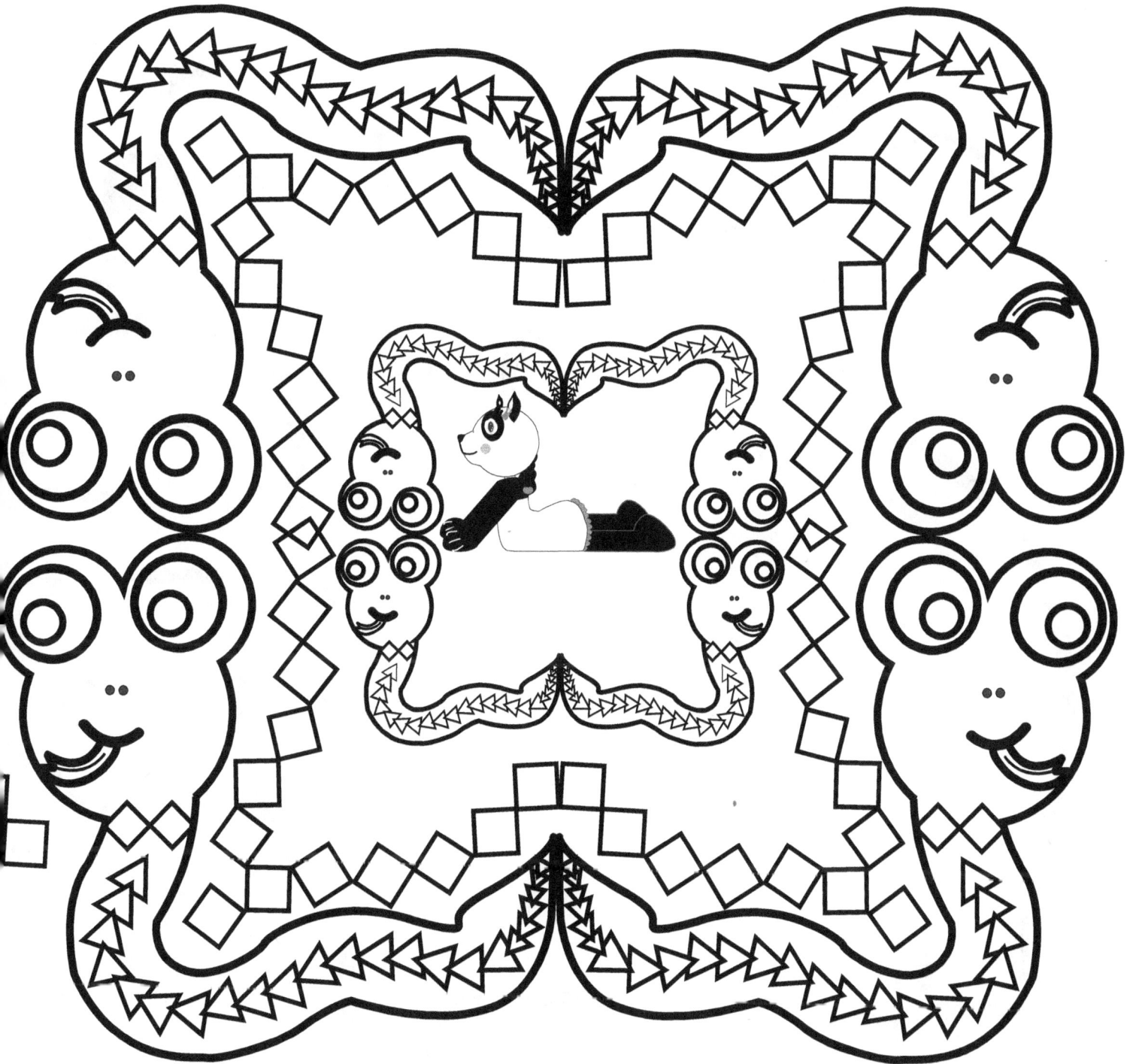

snake - víbora

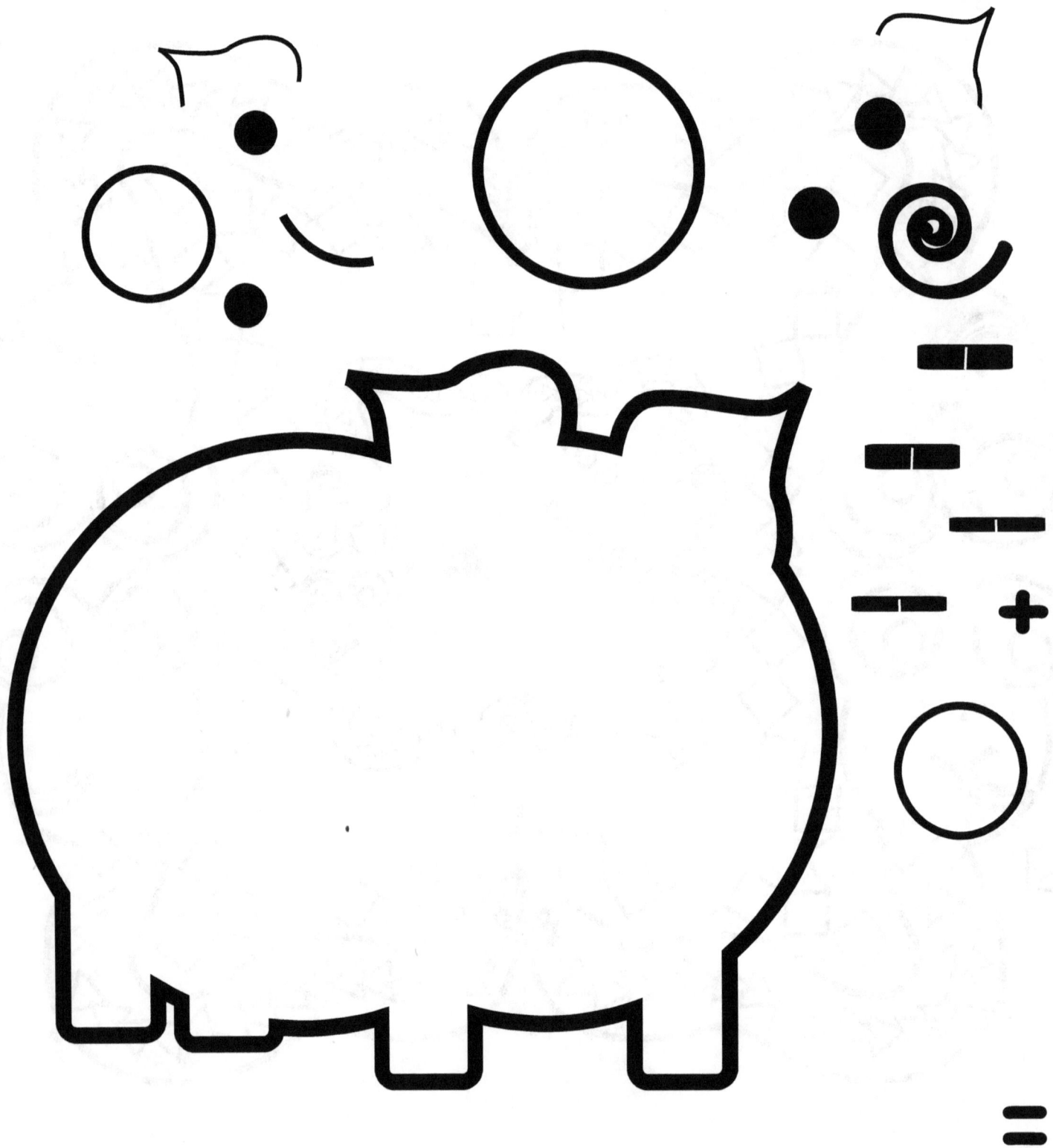

pig - cerdo

Happy Sachi's Yoga

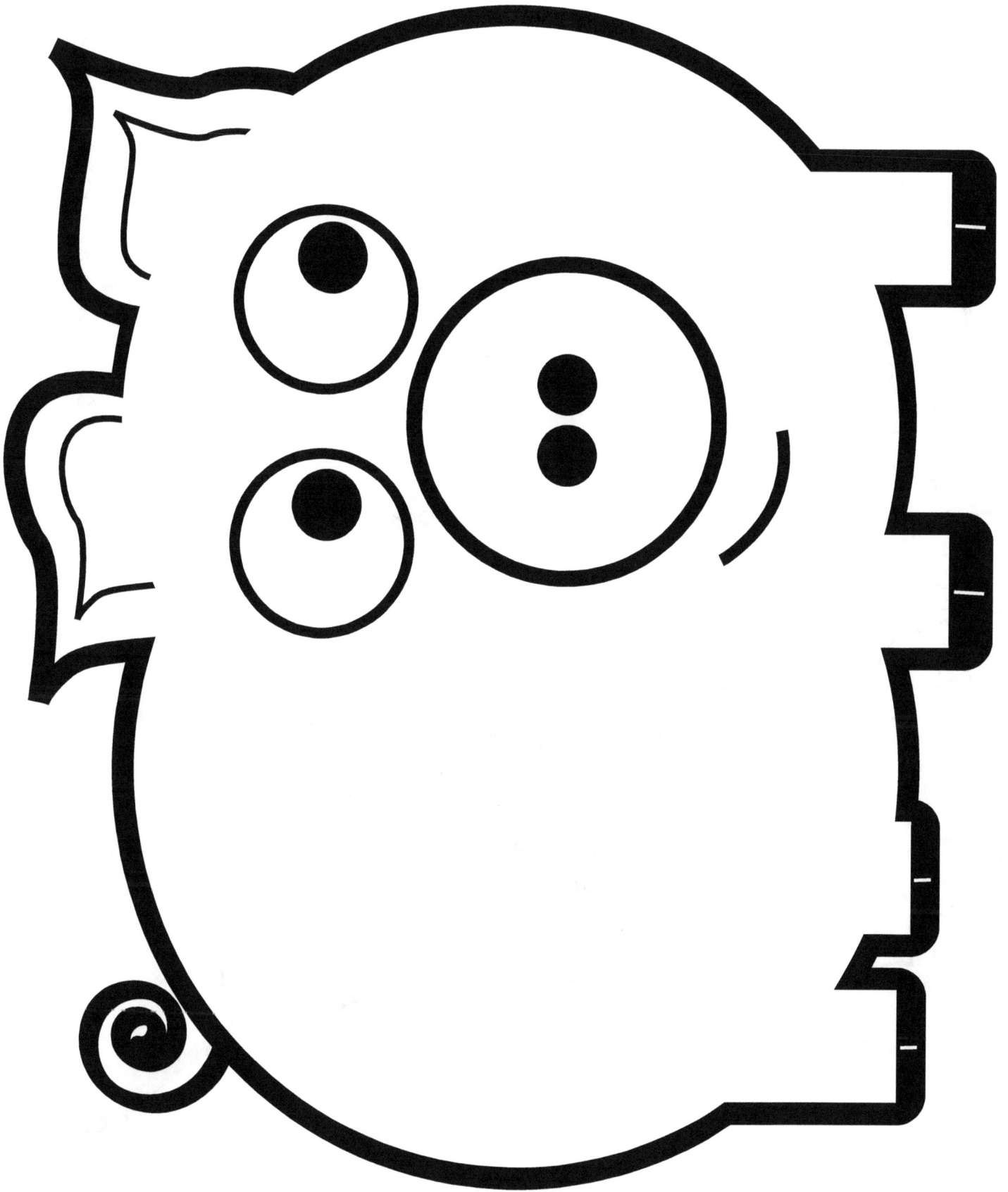

pig - cerdo

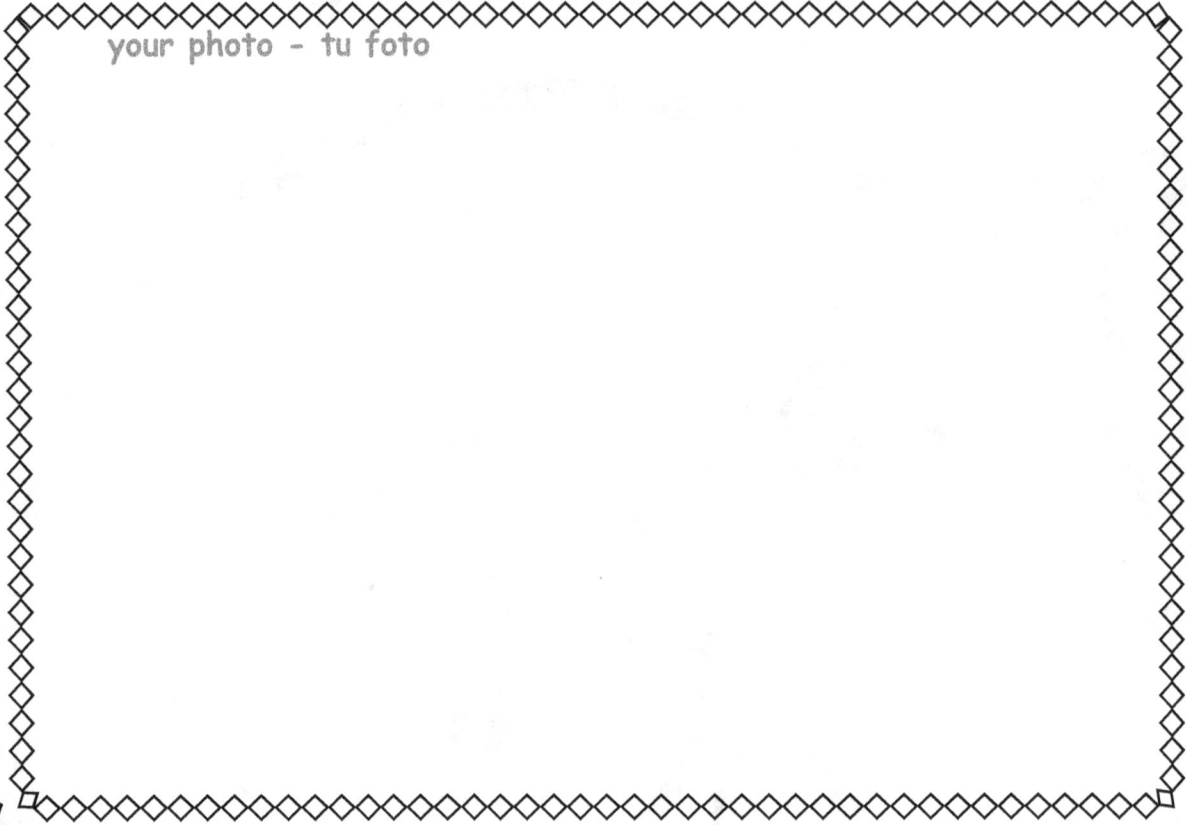

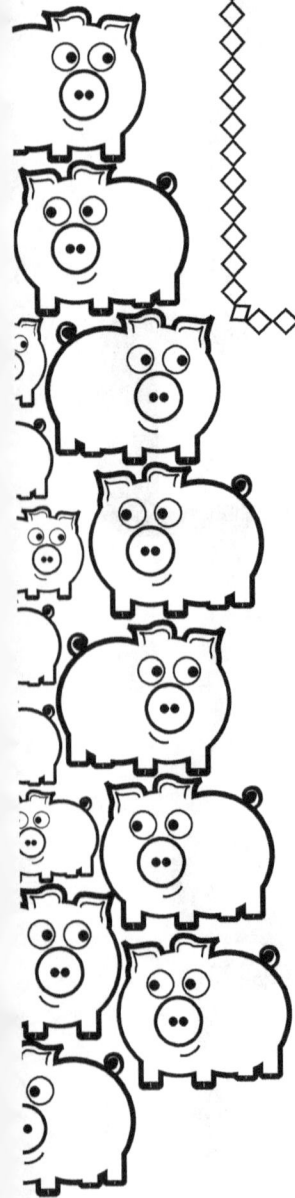

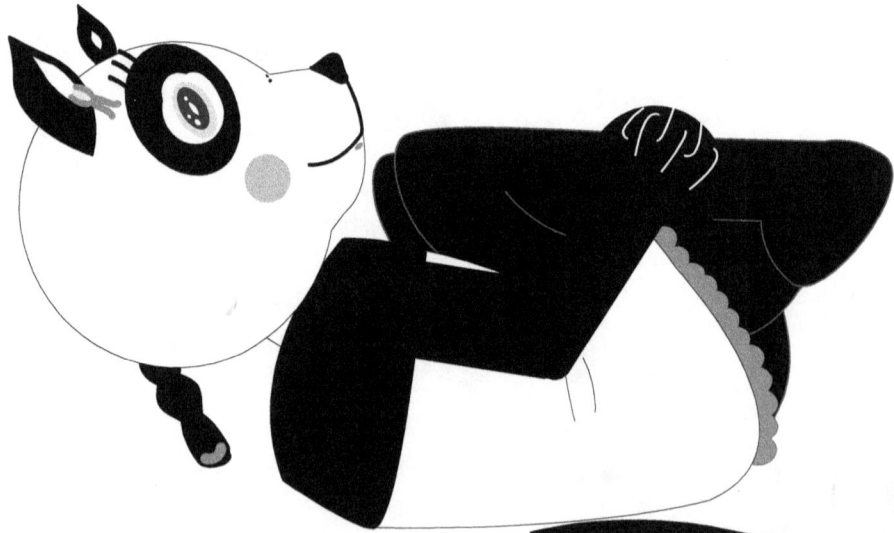

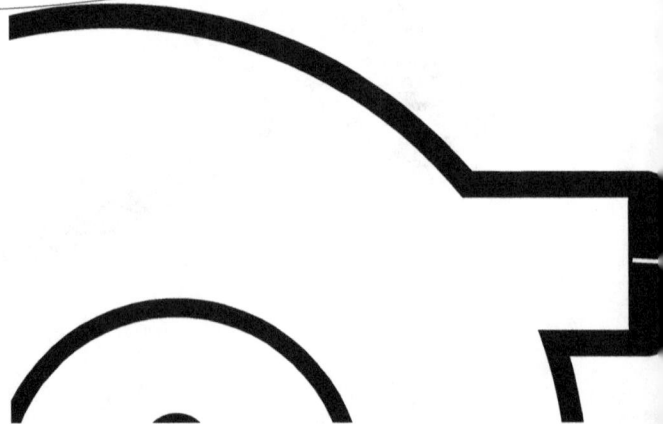

pig - cerdo

Happy Sachi's Yoga

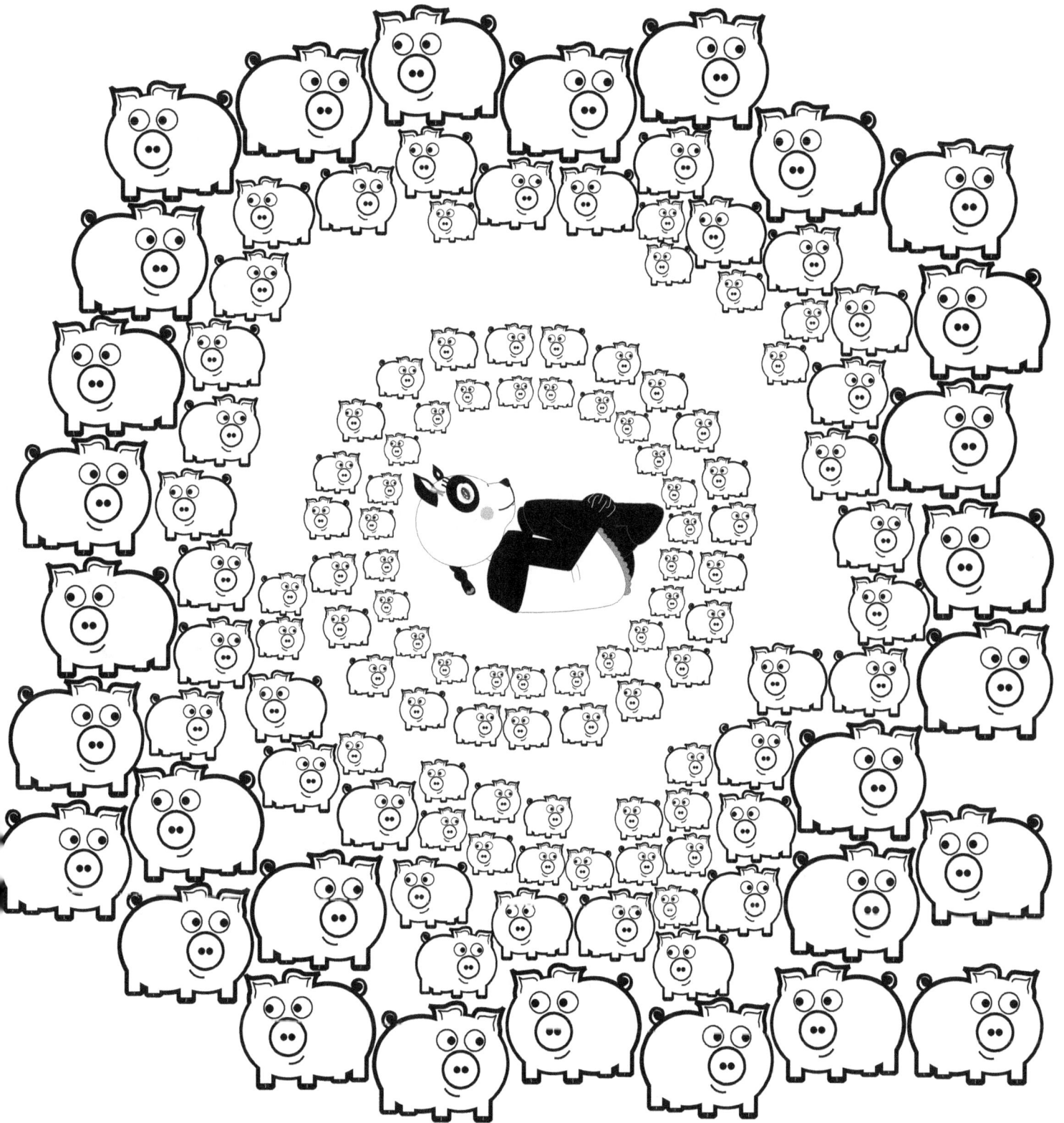

pig - cerdo

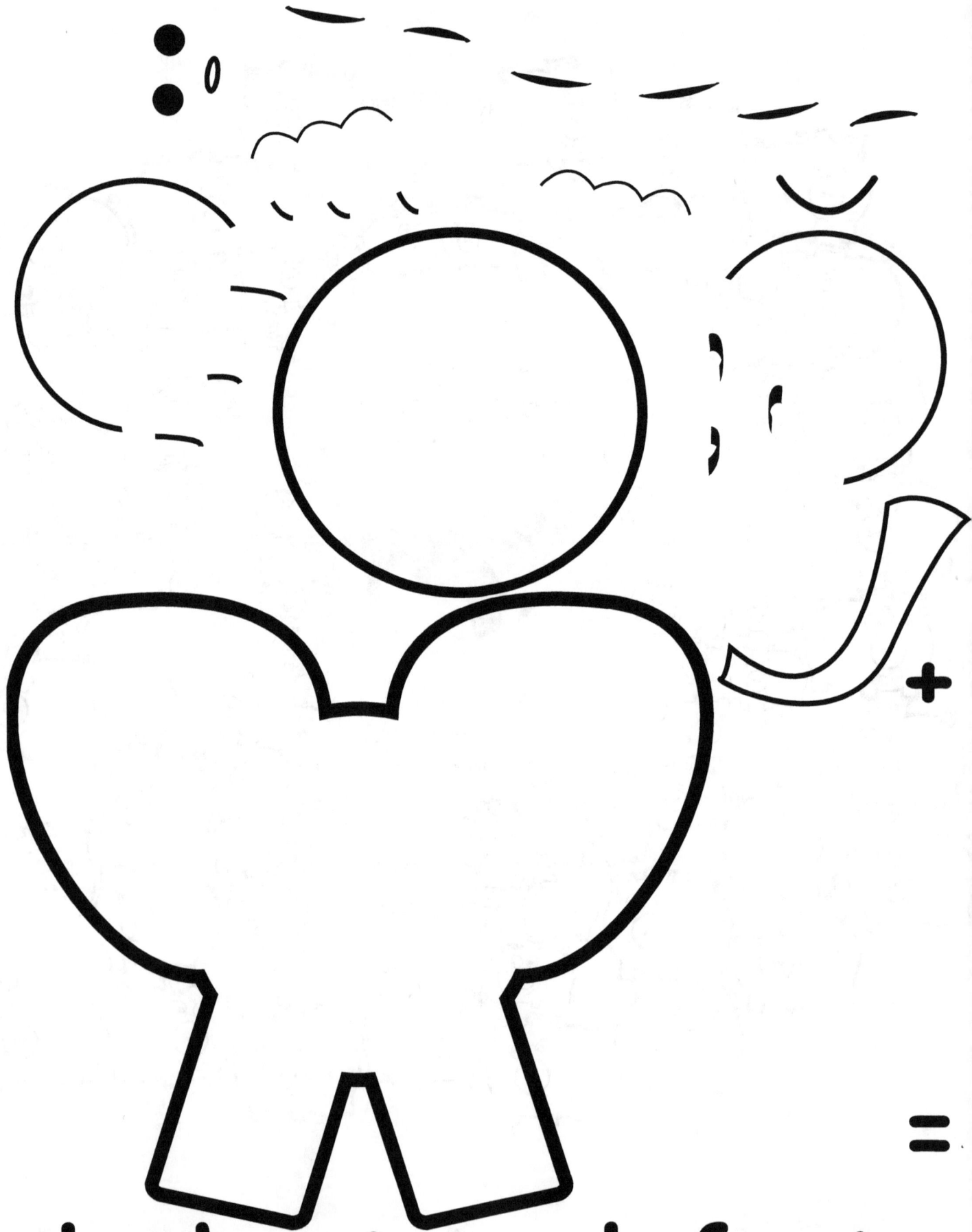

elephant - elefante

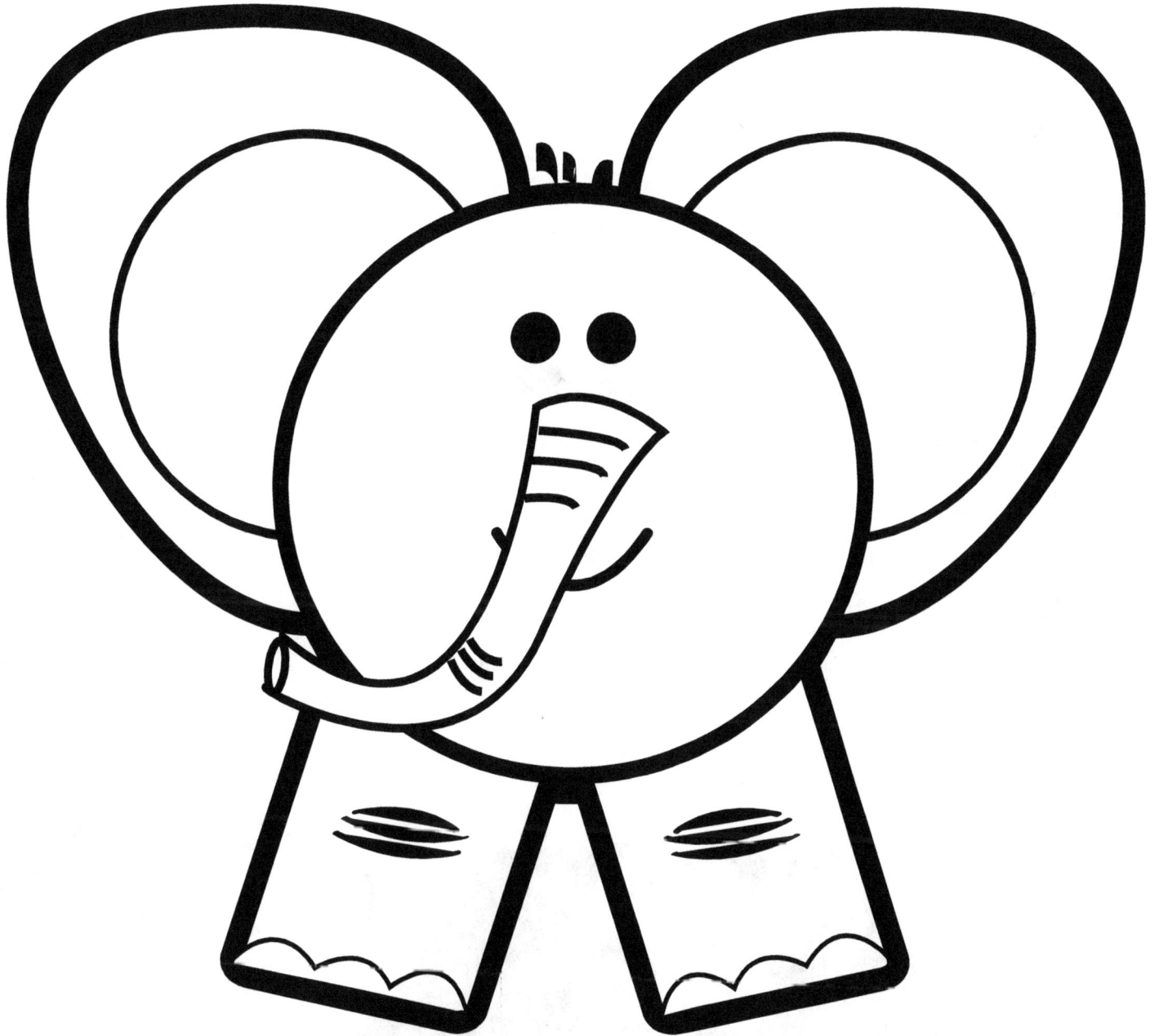

elephant - elefante

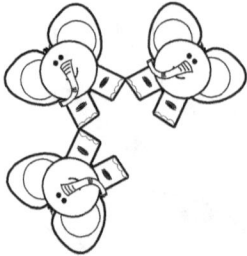

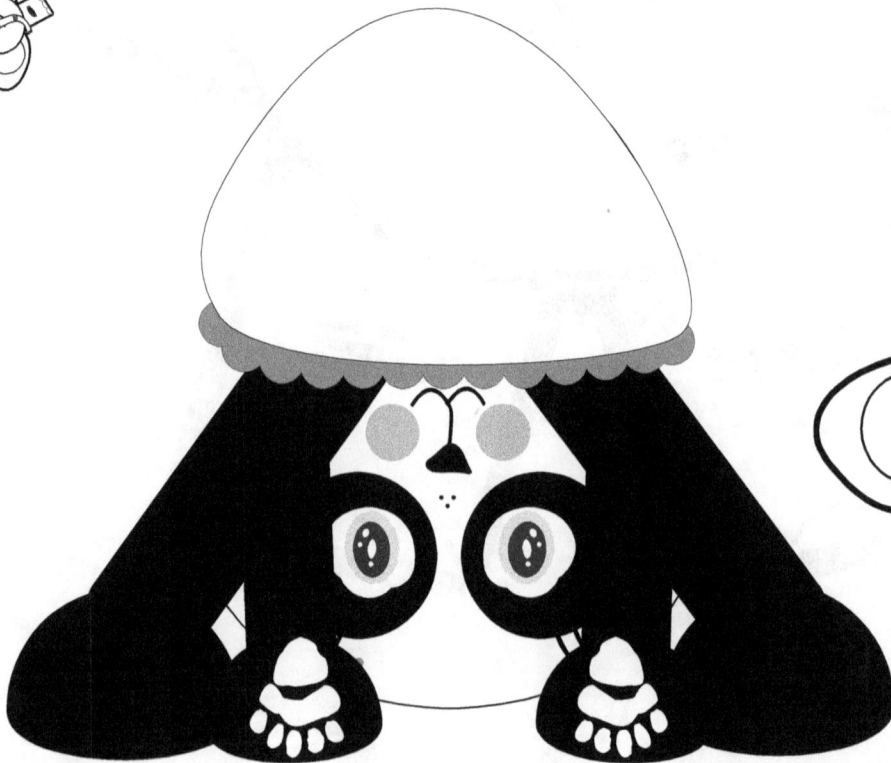

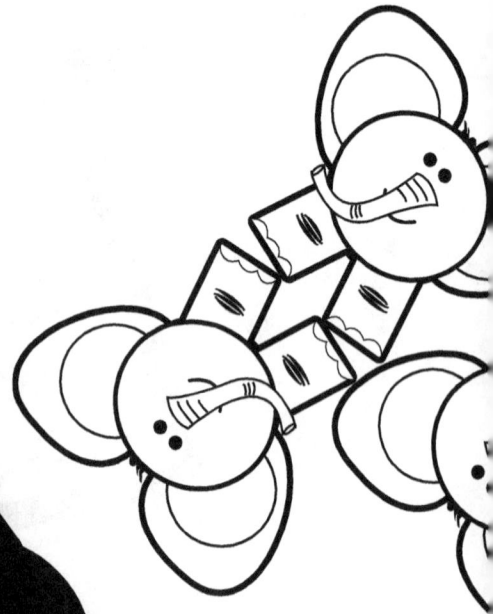

elephant - elefante

Happy Sachi's Yoga

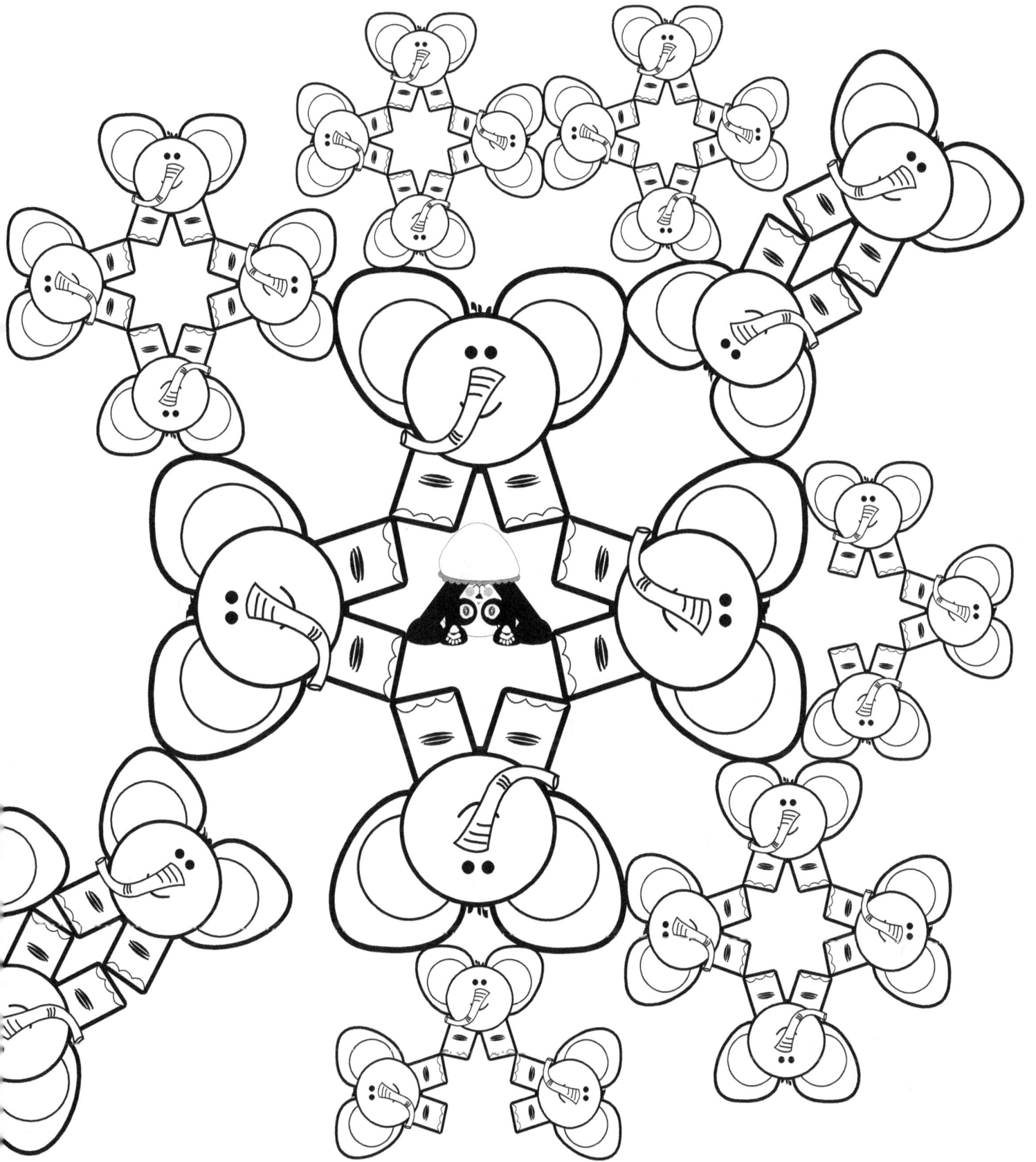

elephant - elefante

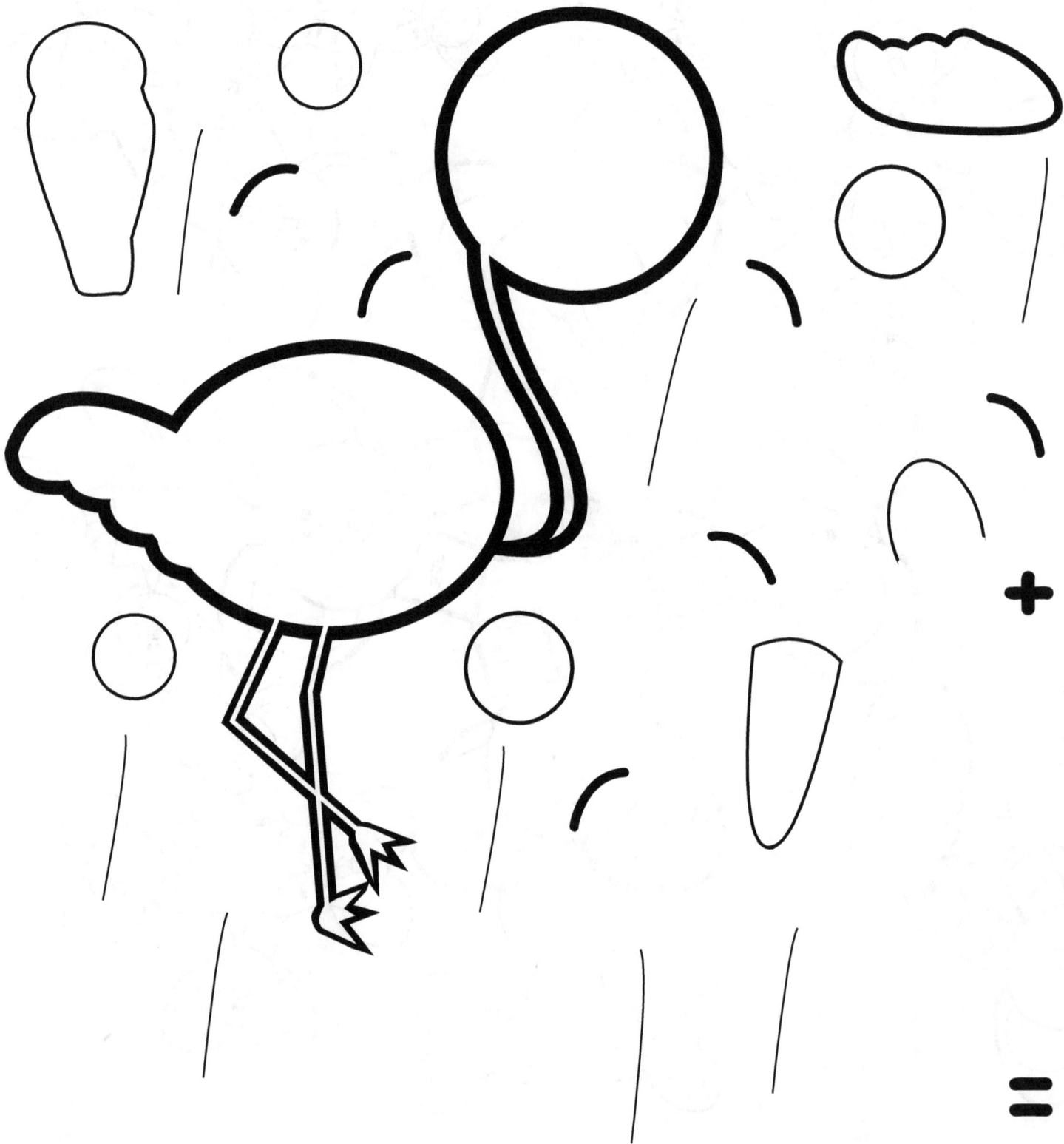

flamingo - flamingo

Happy Sachi's Yoga

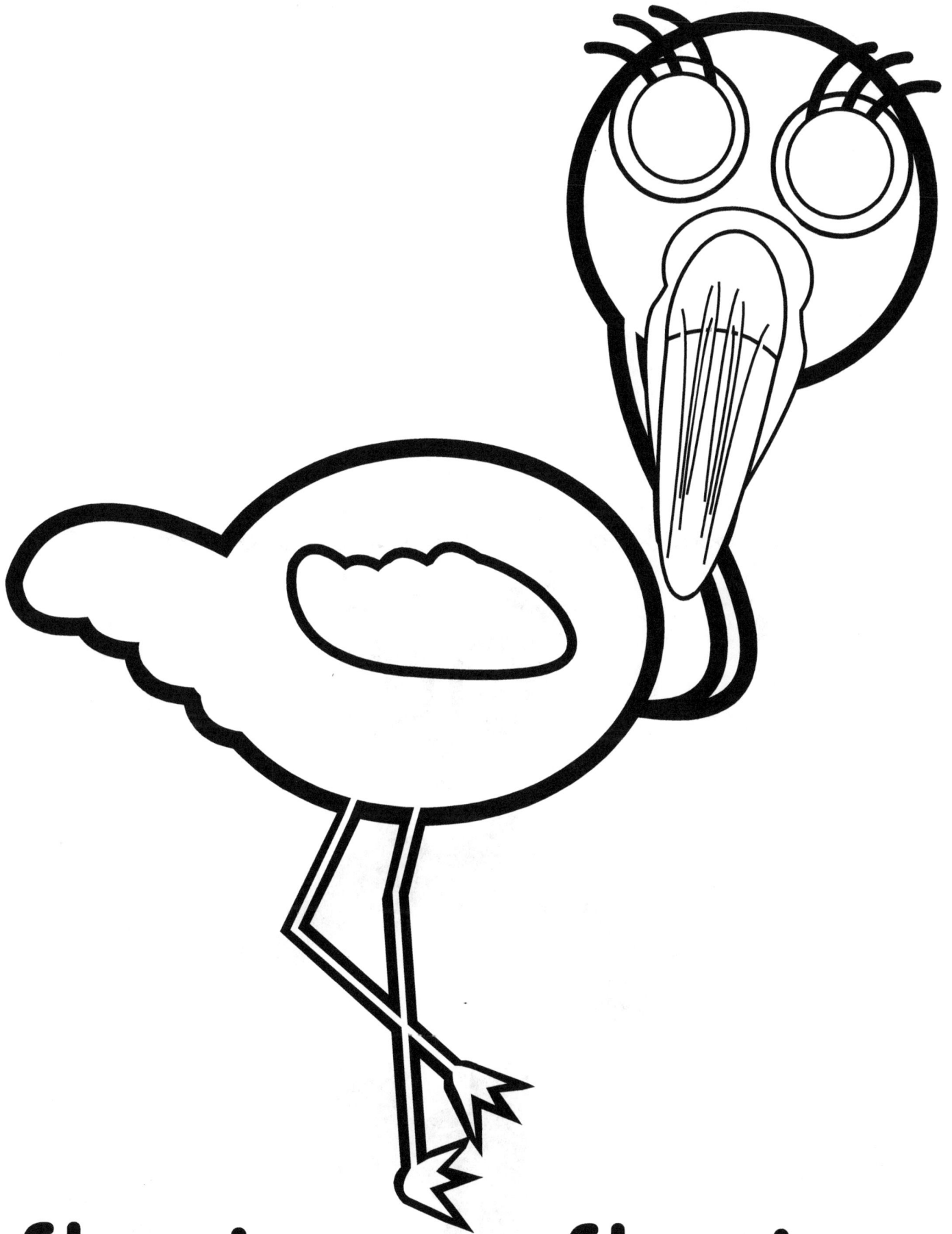

flamingo - flamingo

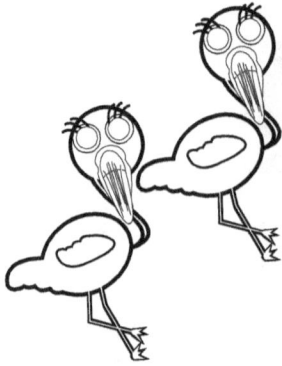

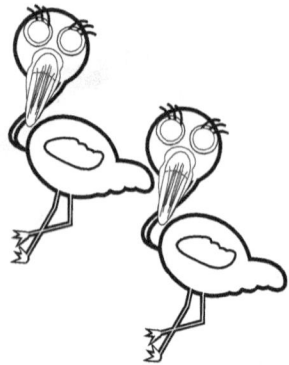

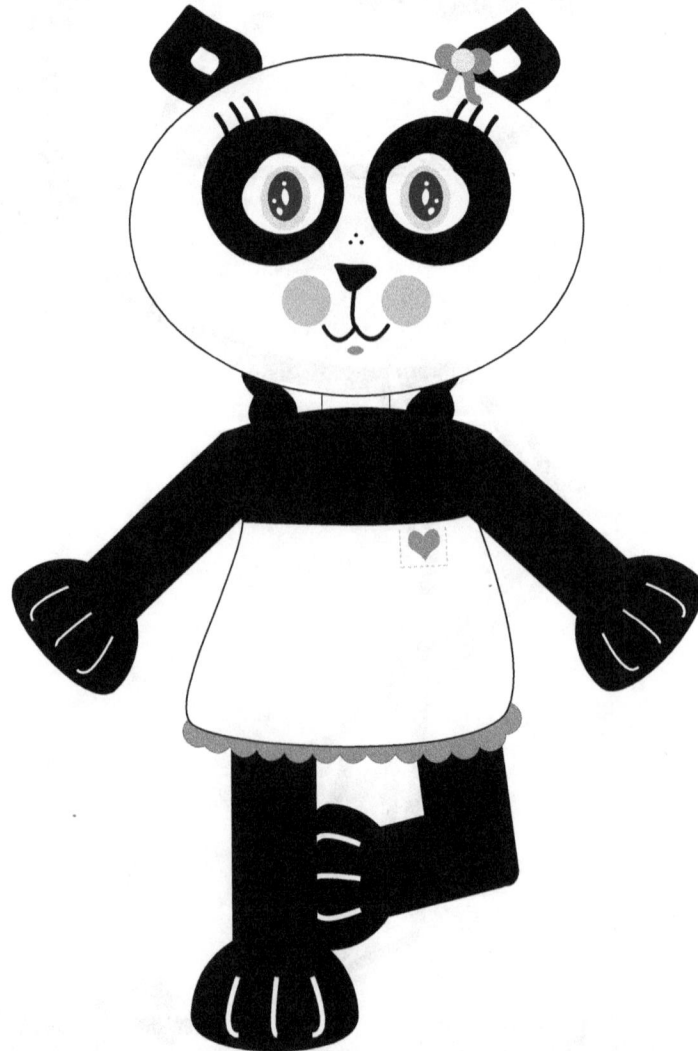

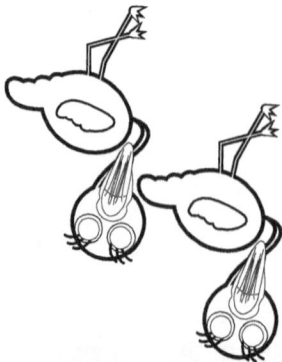

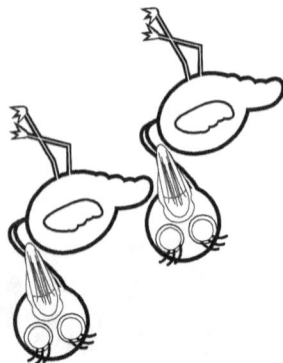

flamingo - flamingo

Happy Sachi's Yoga

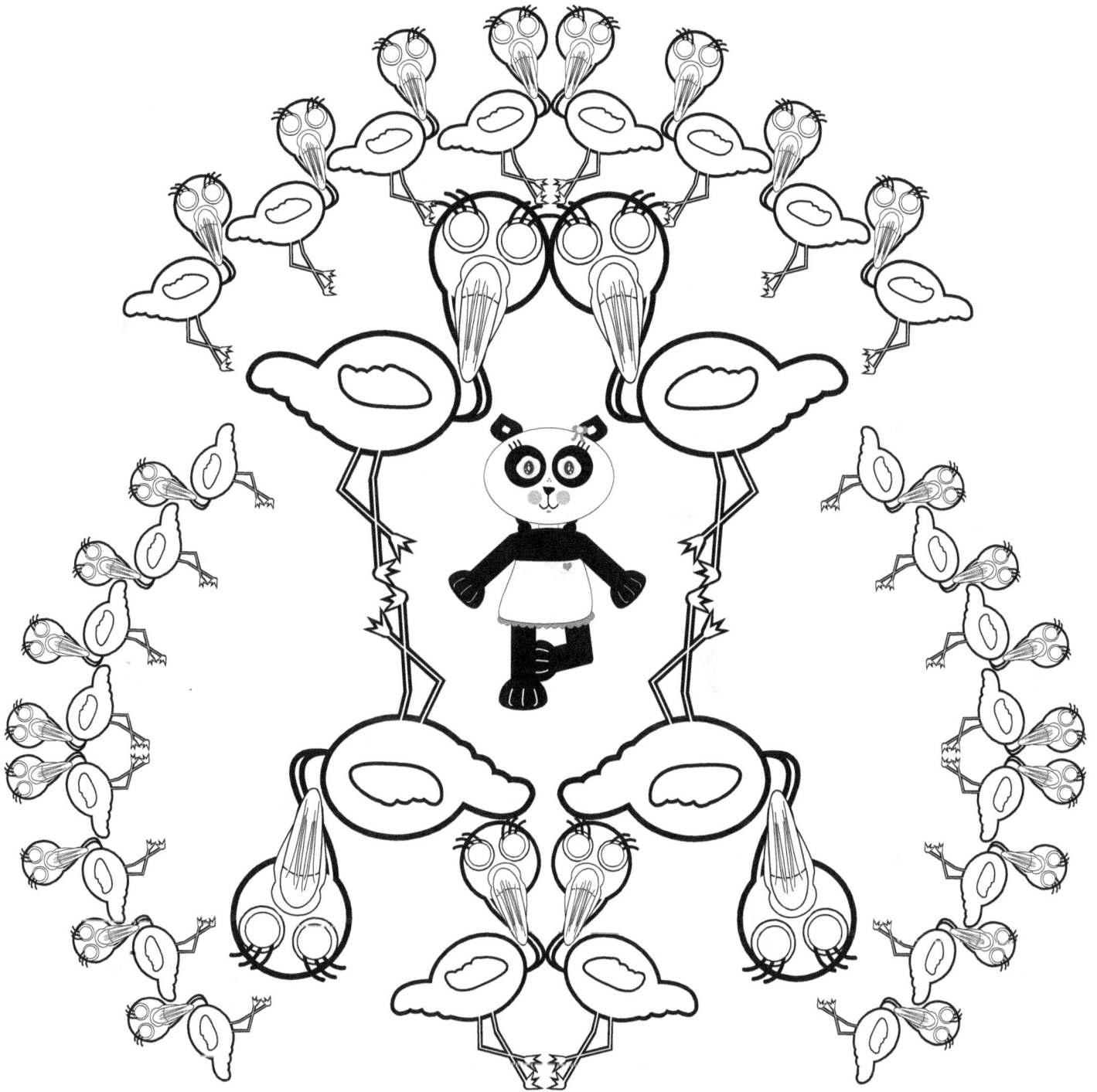

flamingo - flamingo

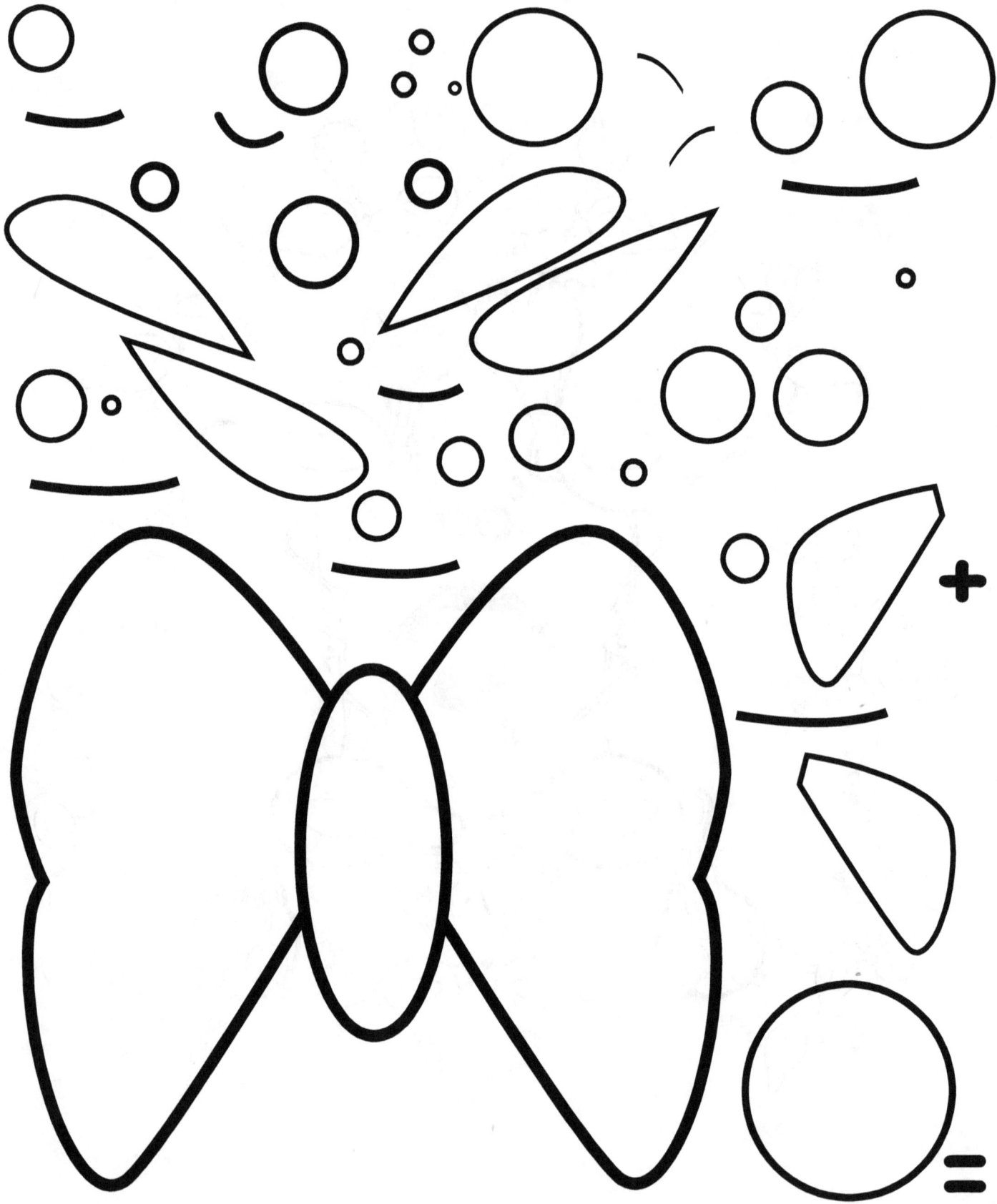

butterfly - mariposa

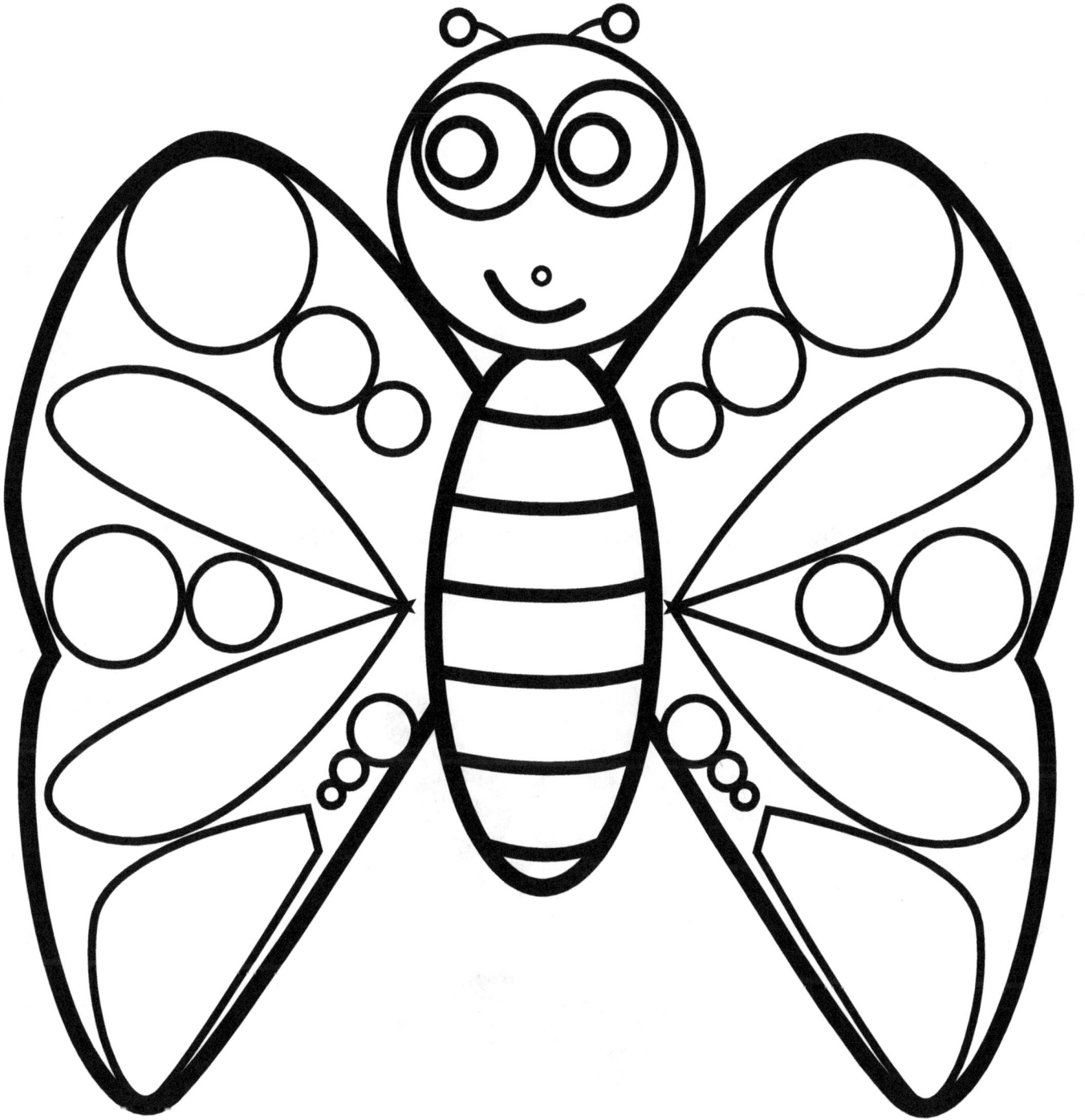

butterfly - mariposa

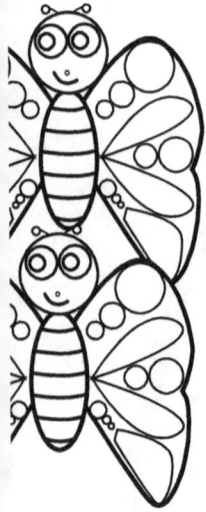

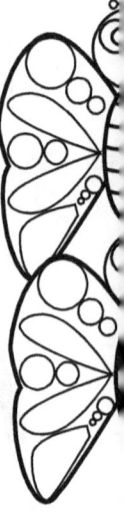

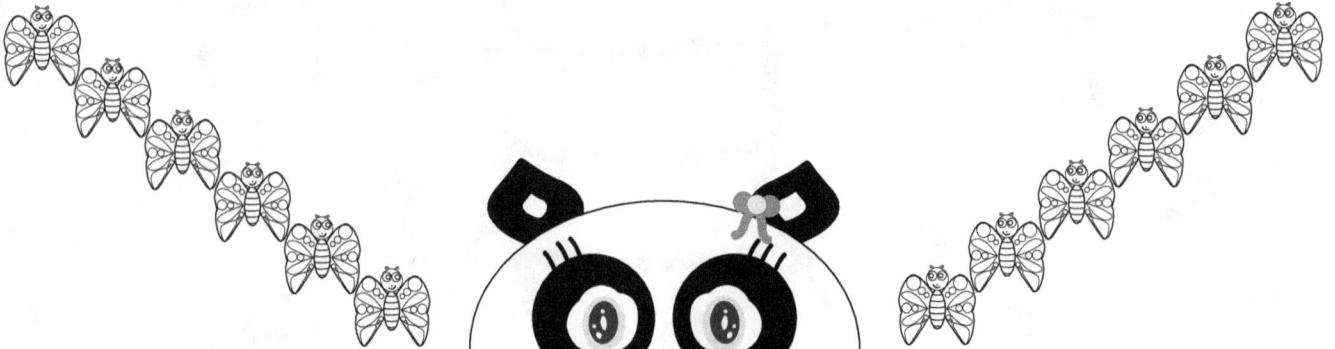

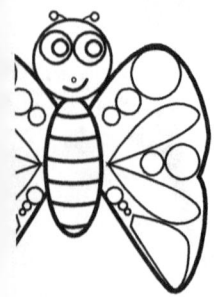

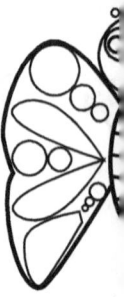

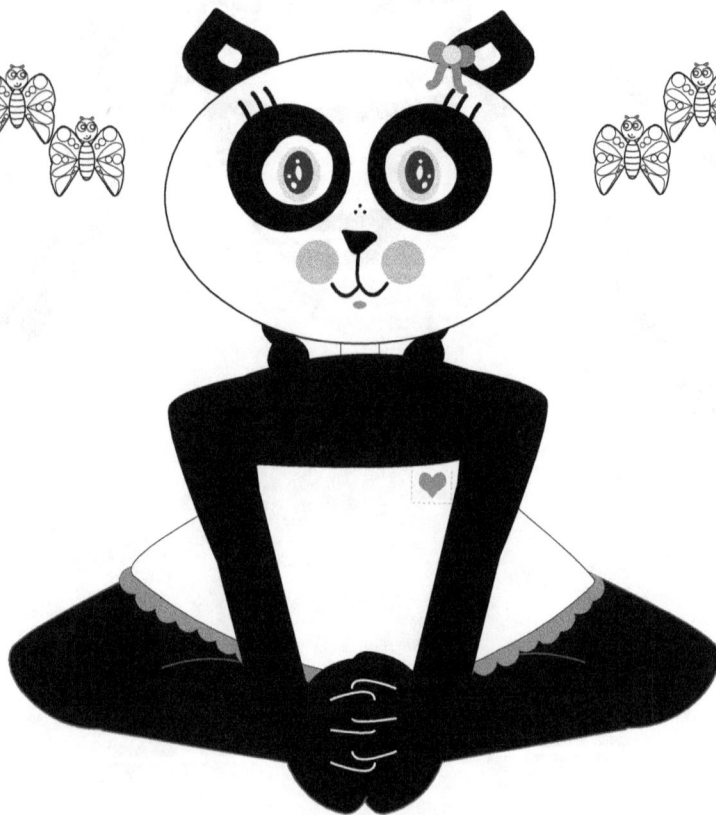

butterfly - mariposa

Happy Sachi's Yoga

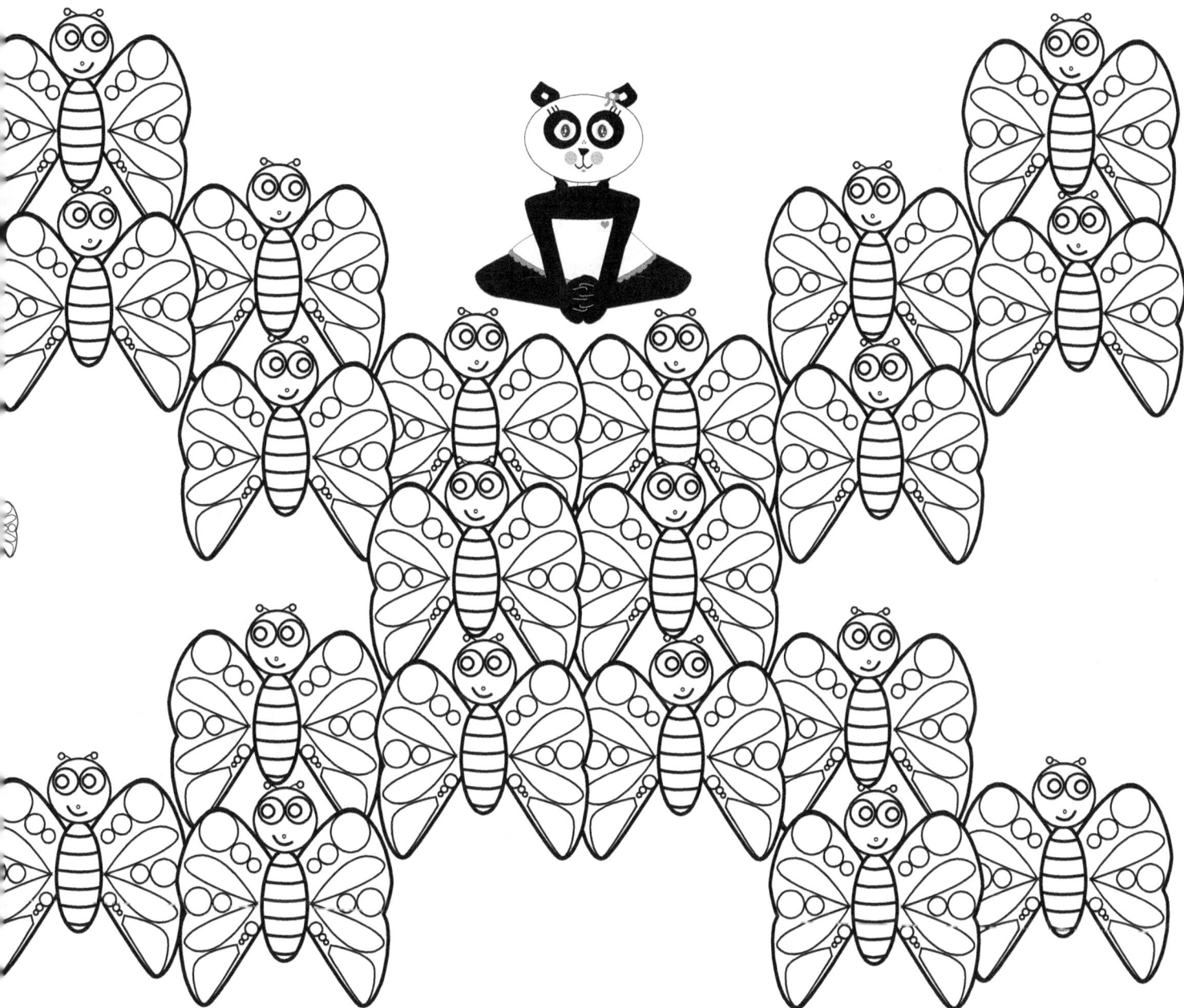

butterfly - mariposa

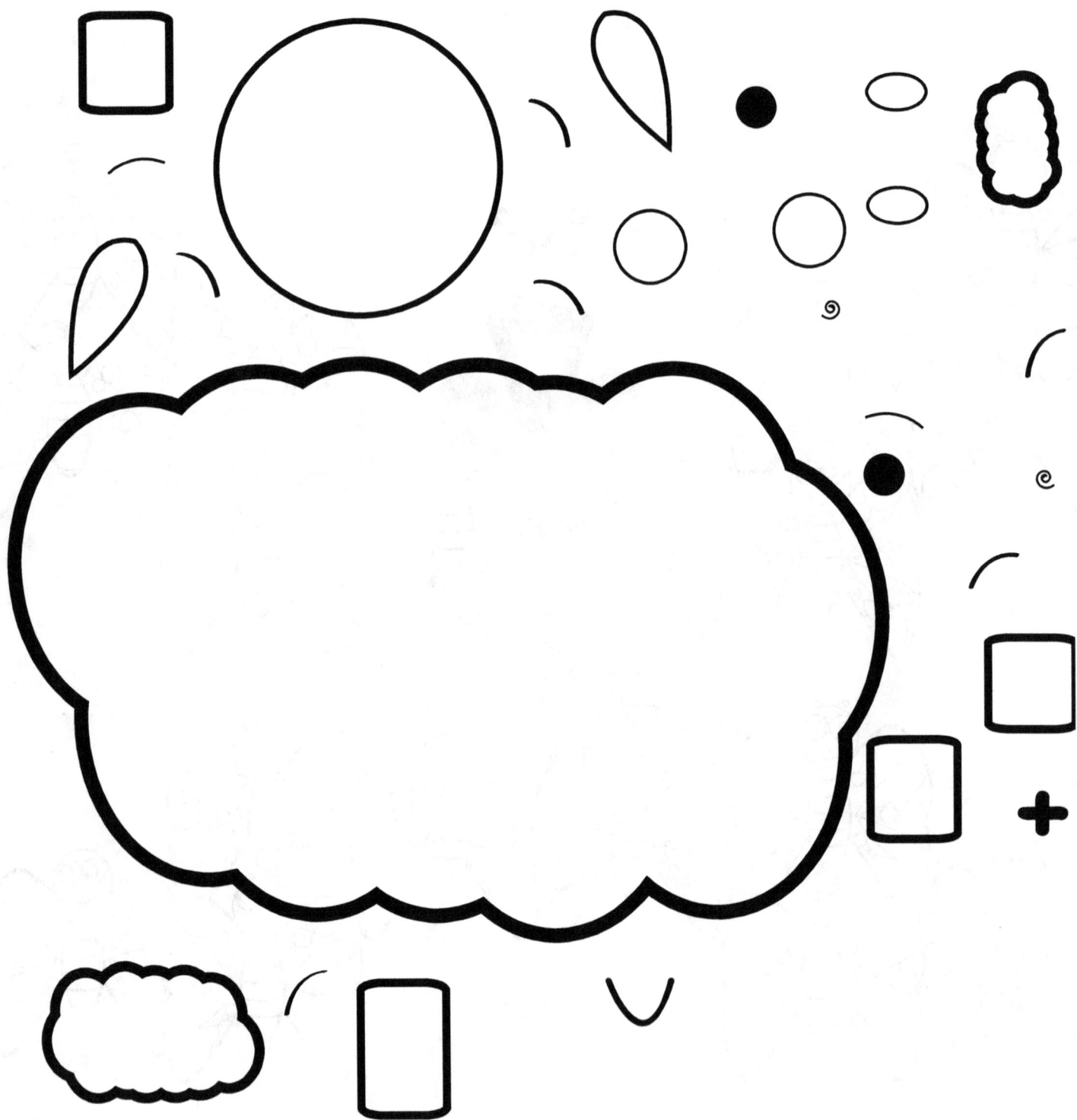

sheep - borrego

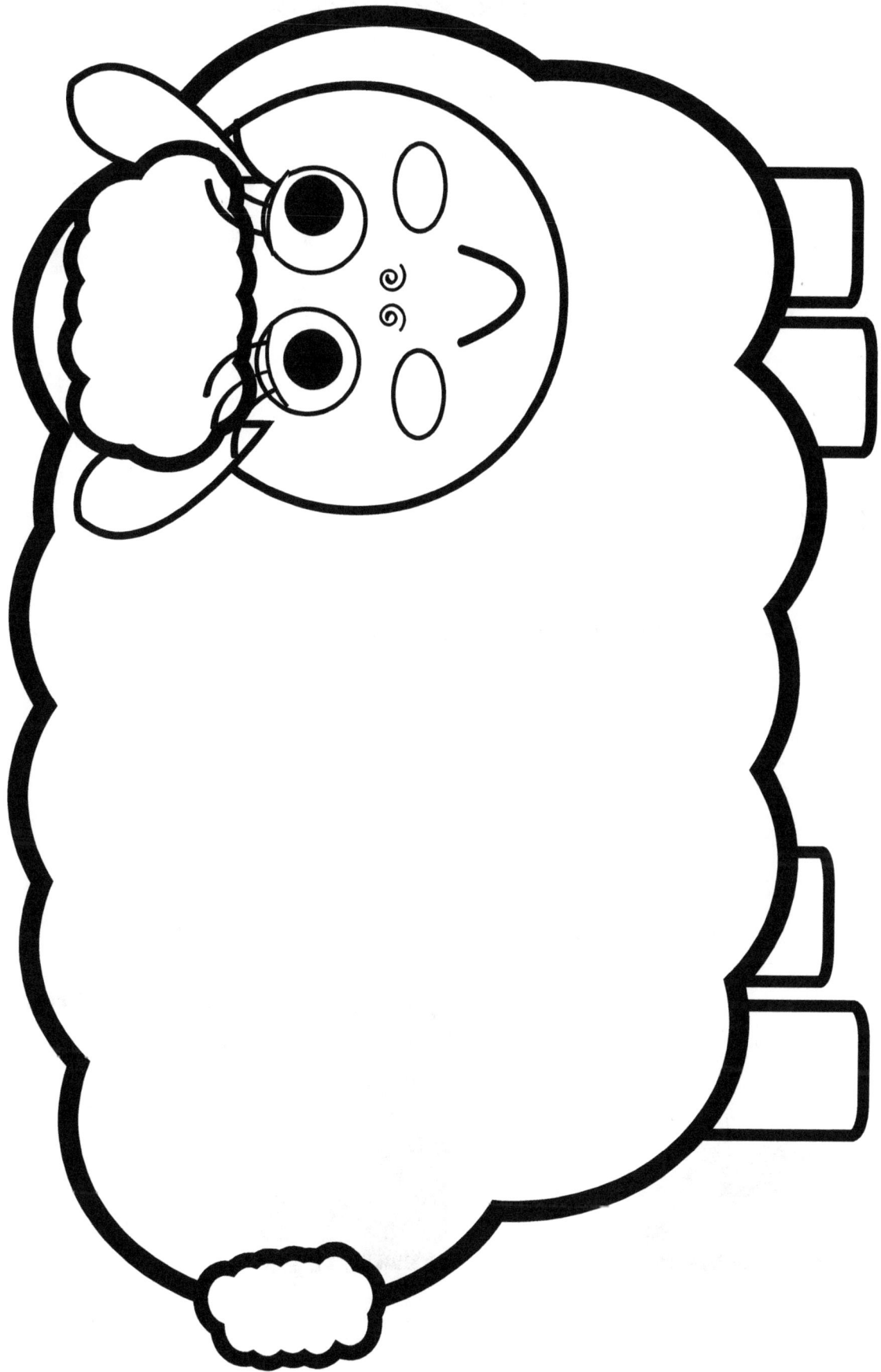

sheep - borrego

your photo - tu foto

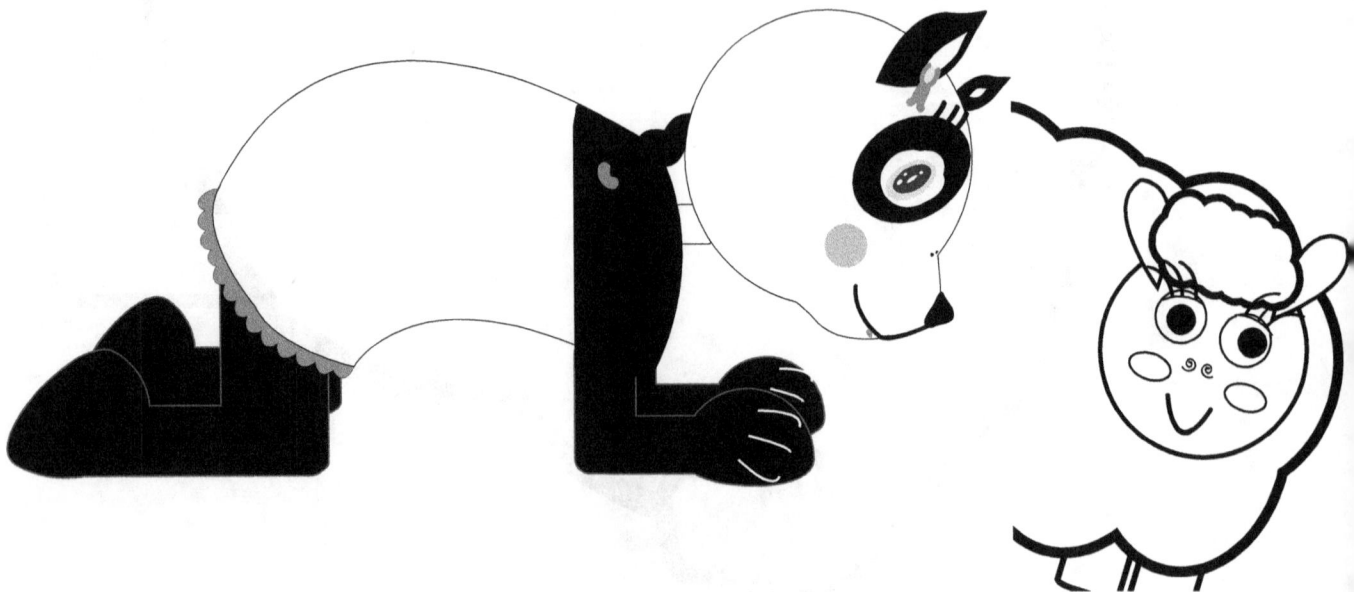

sheep - borrego

Happy Sachi's Yoga

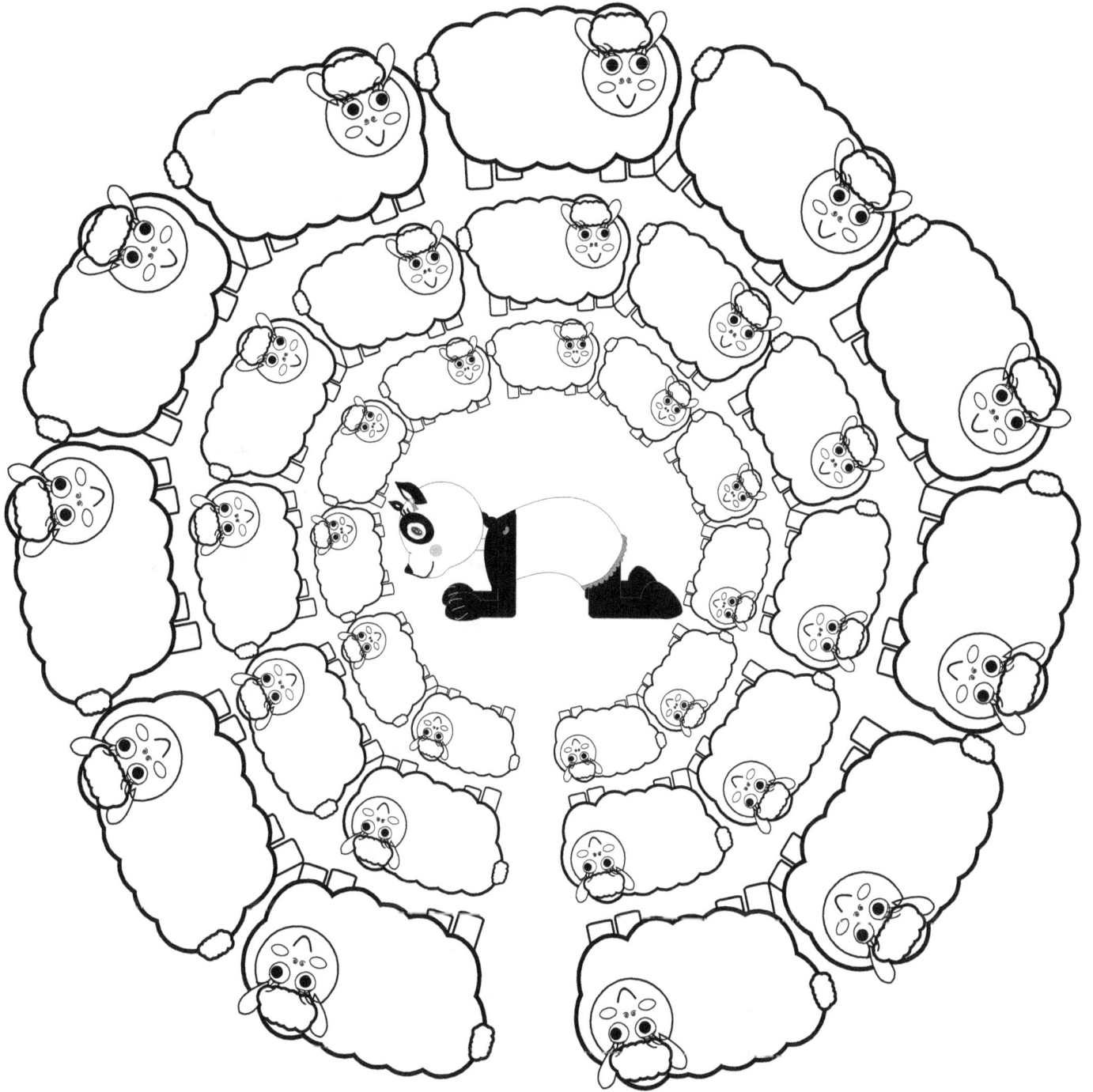

sheep - borrego

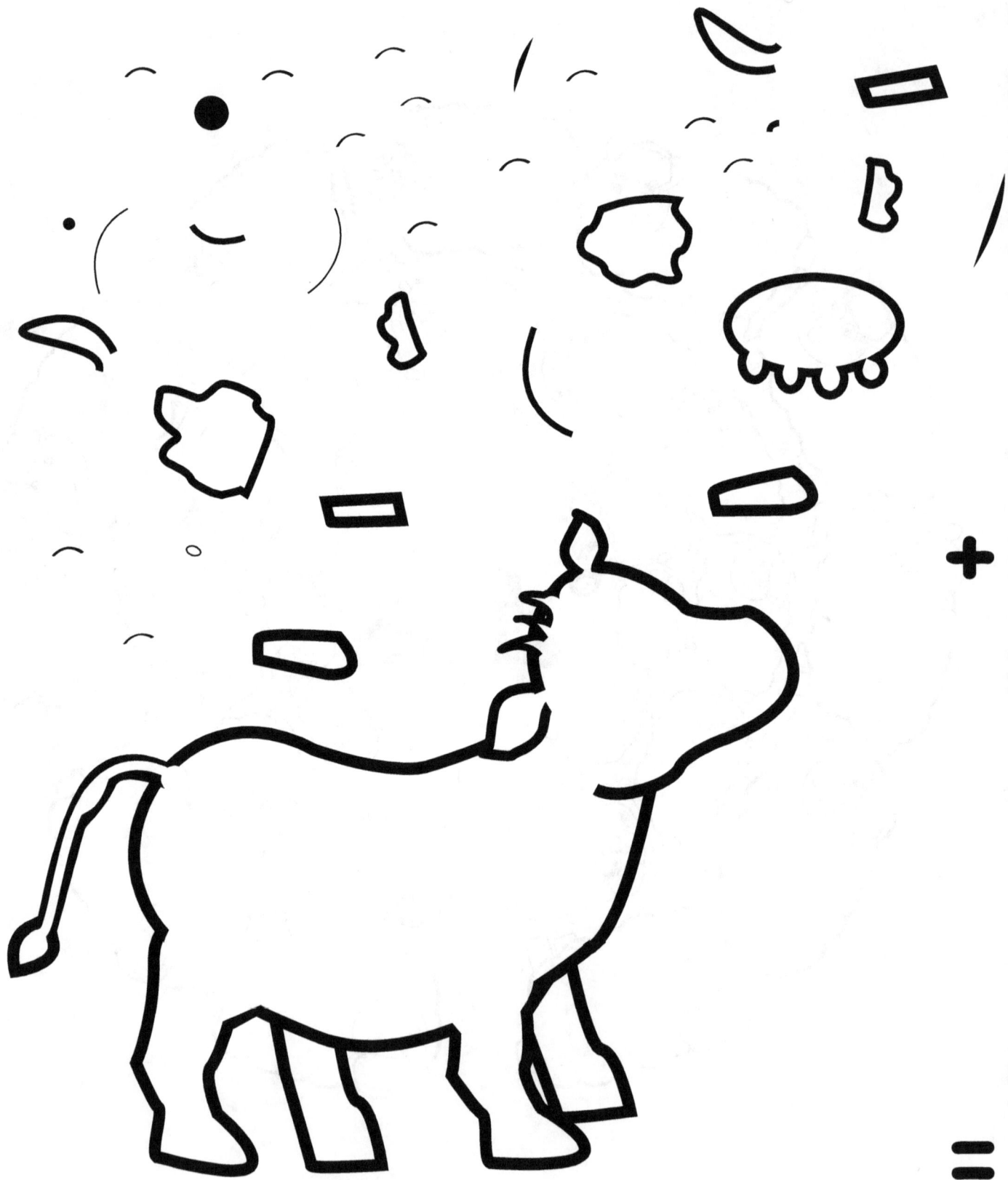

cow - vaca

Happy Sachi's Yoga

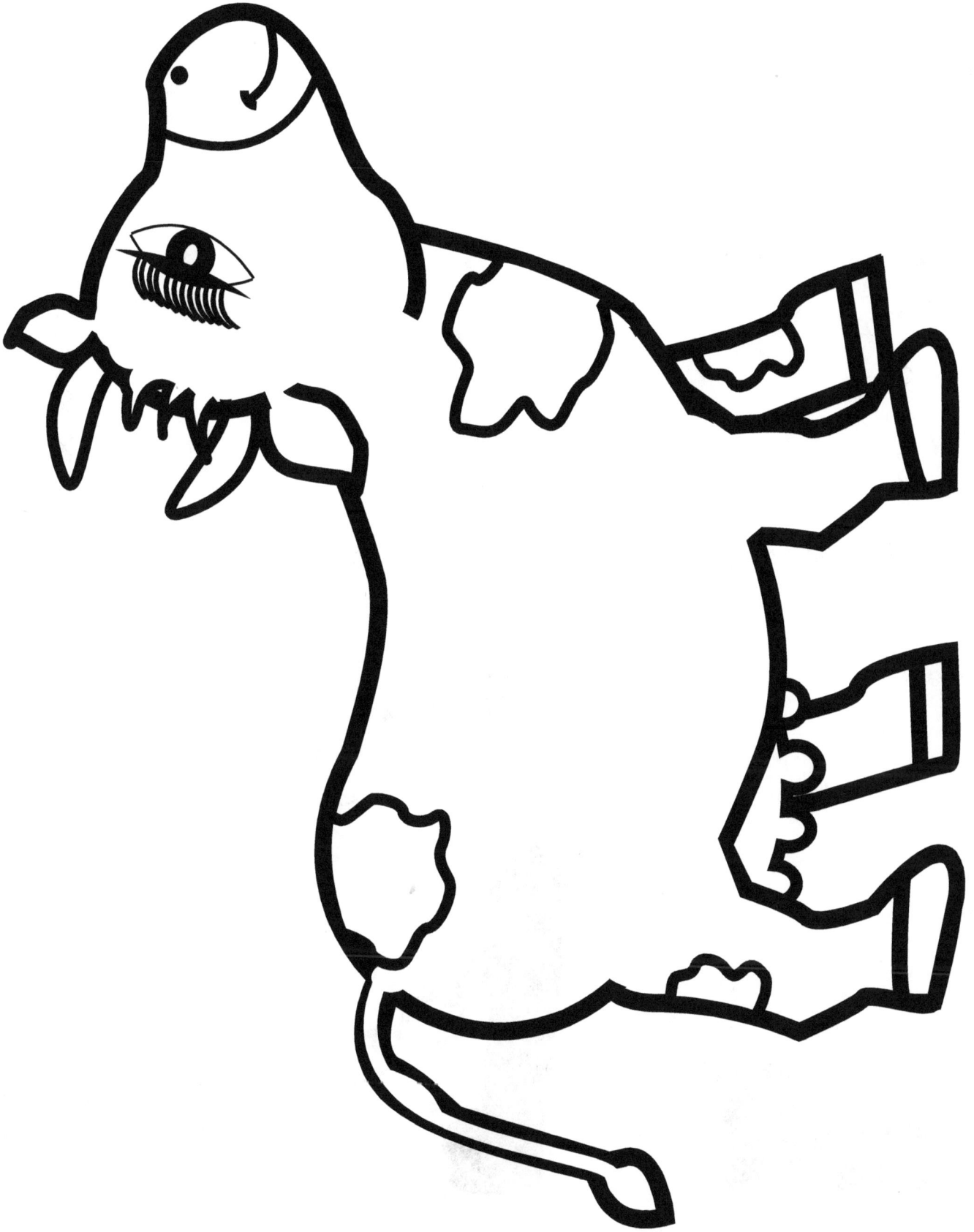

cow - vaca

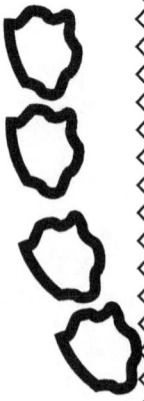

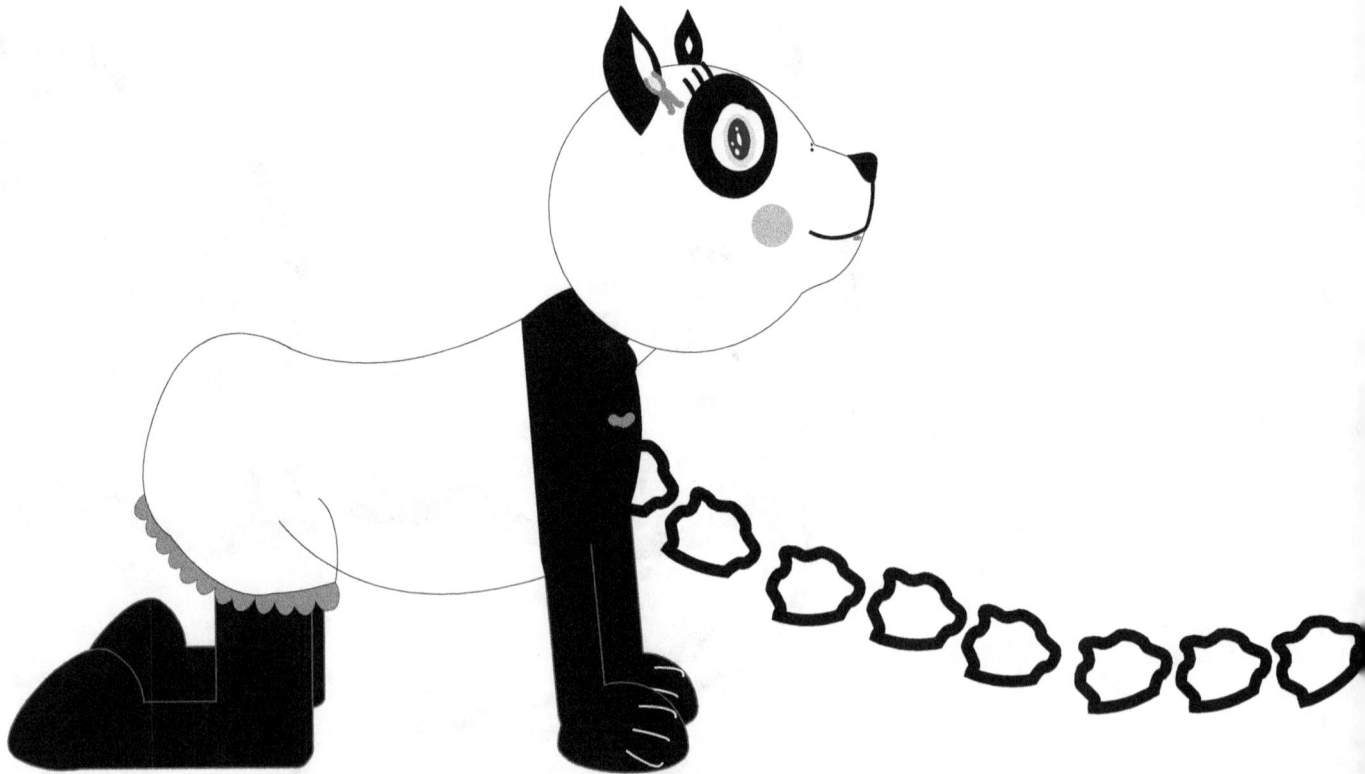

cow - vaca

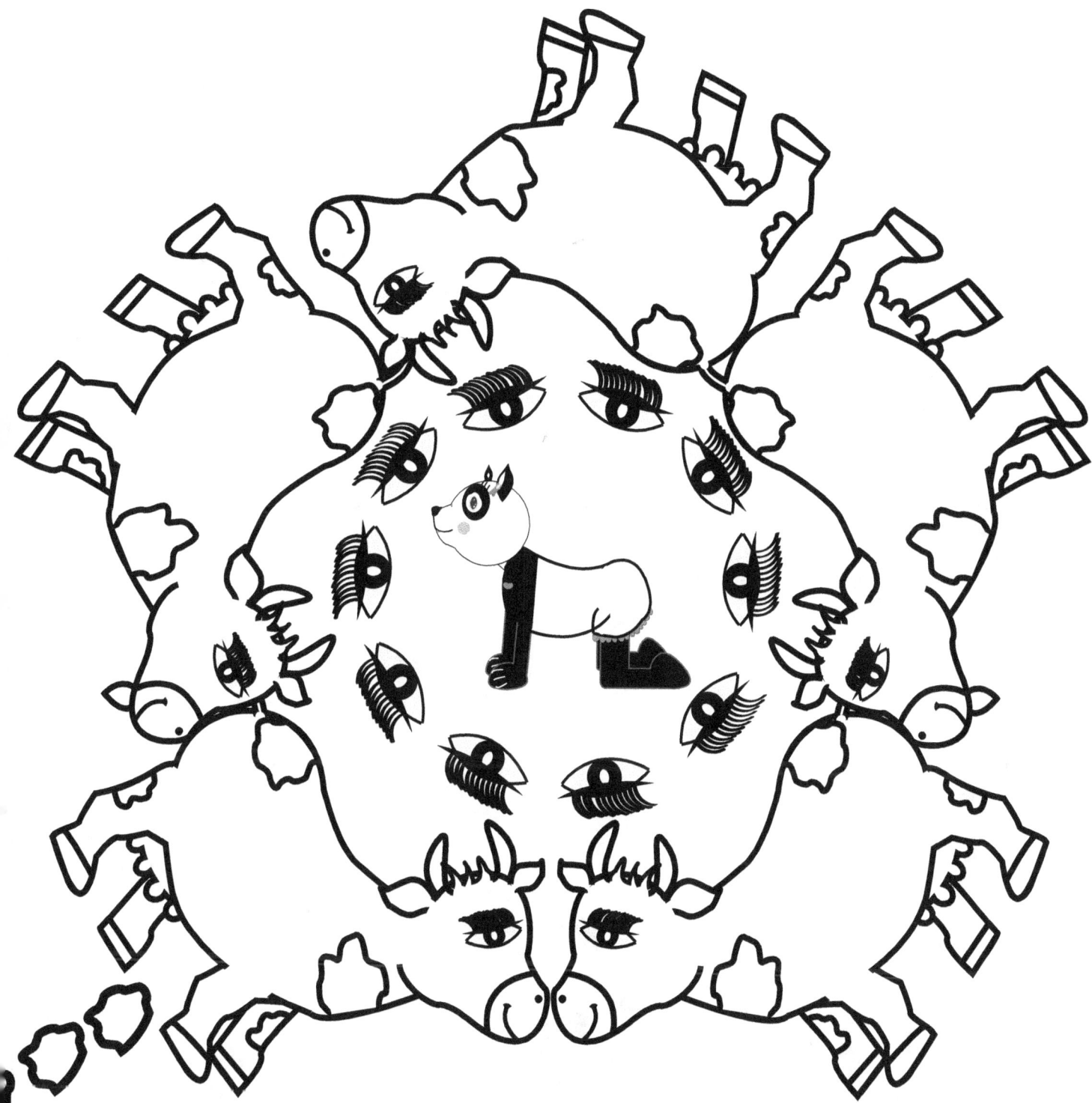

cow - vaca

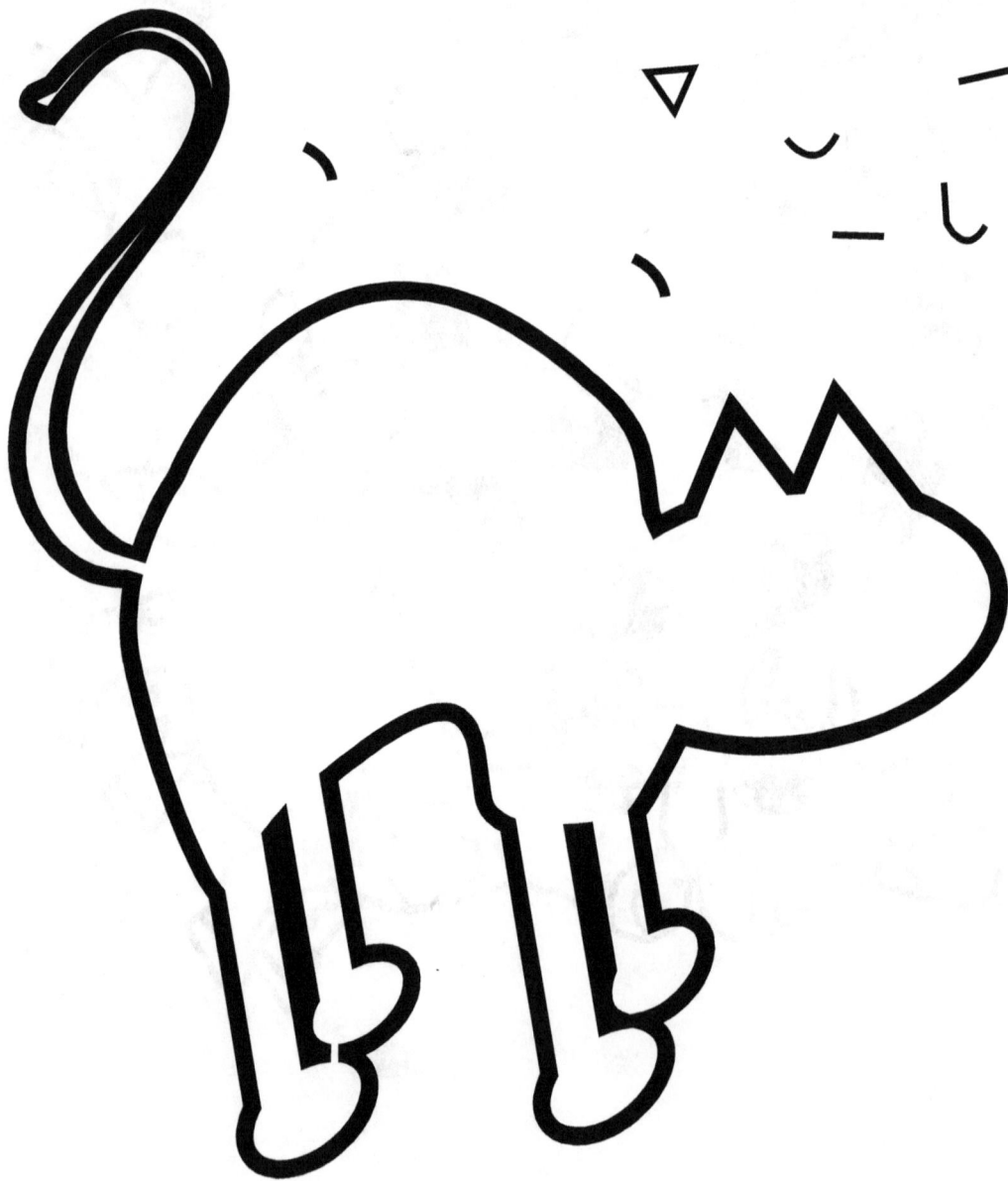

cat - gato

Happy Sachi's Yoga

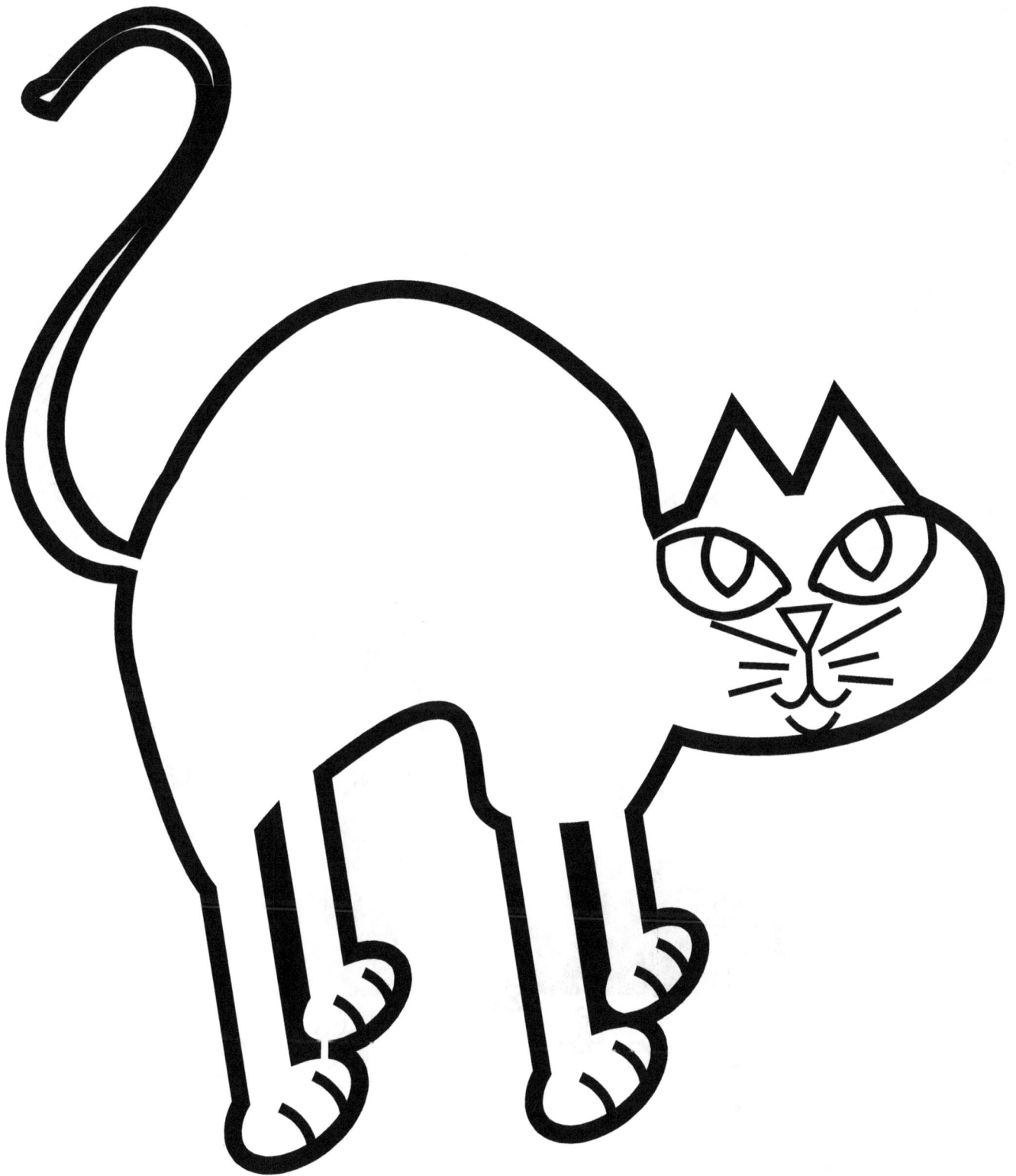

cat - gato

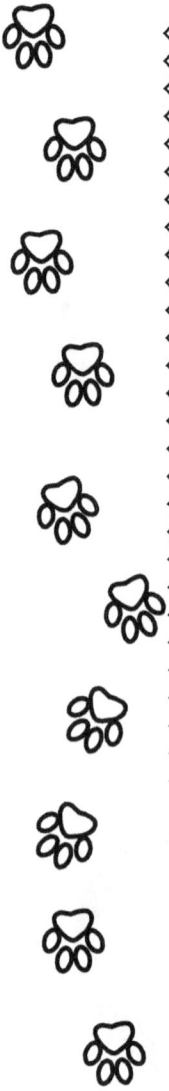

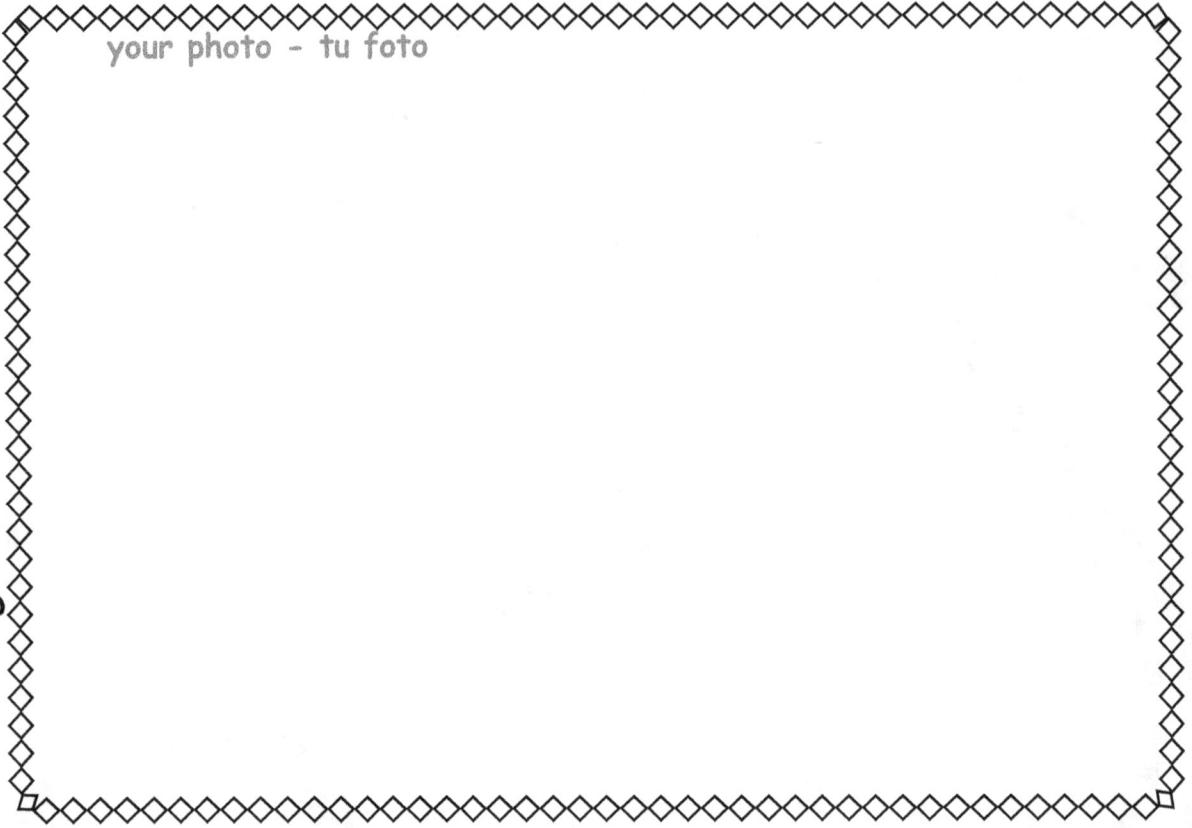

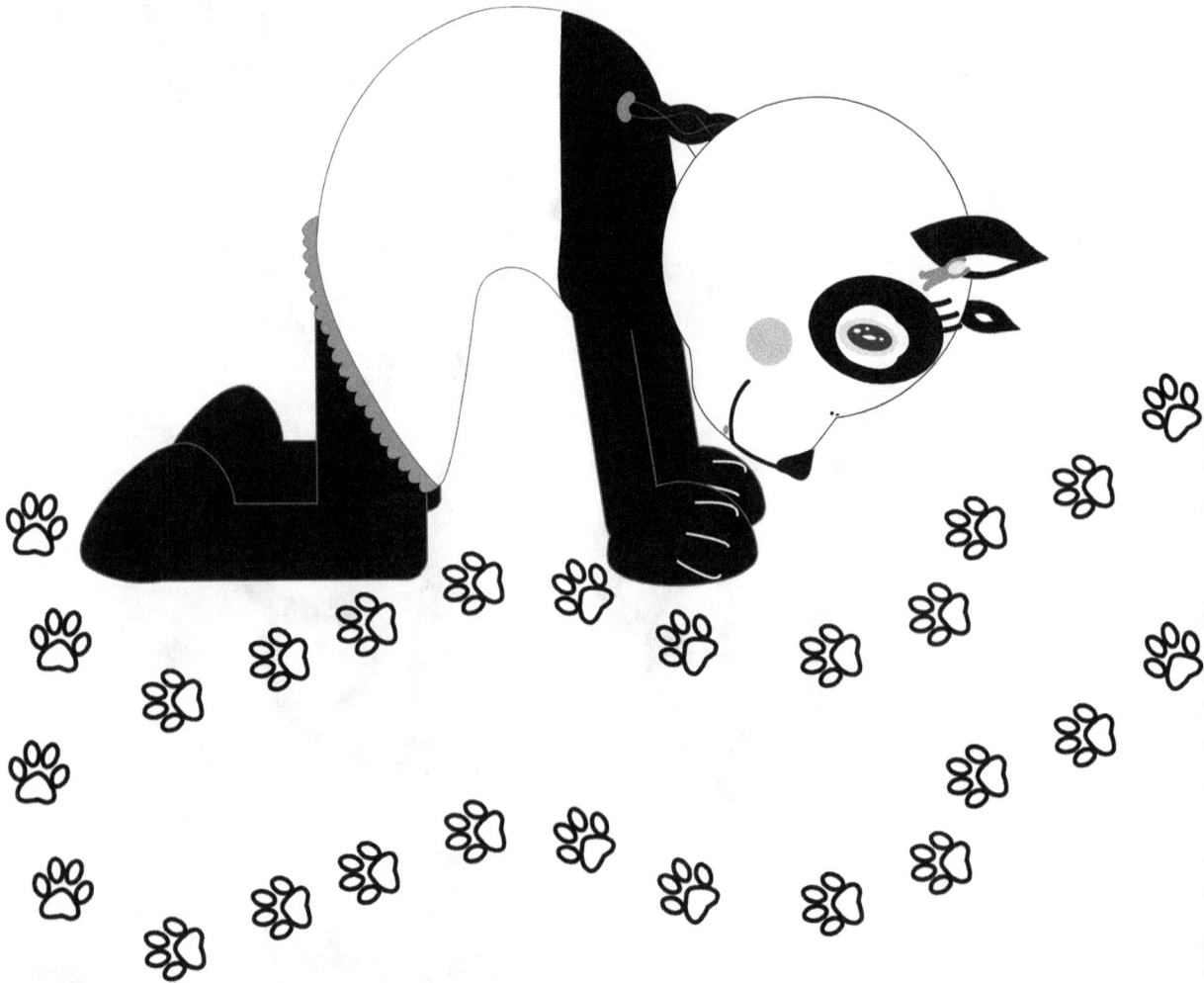

cat - gato

Happy Sachi's Yoga

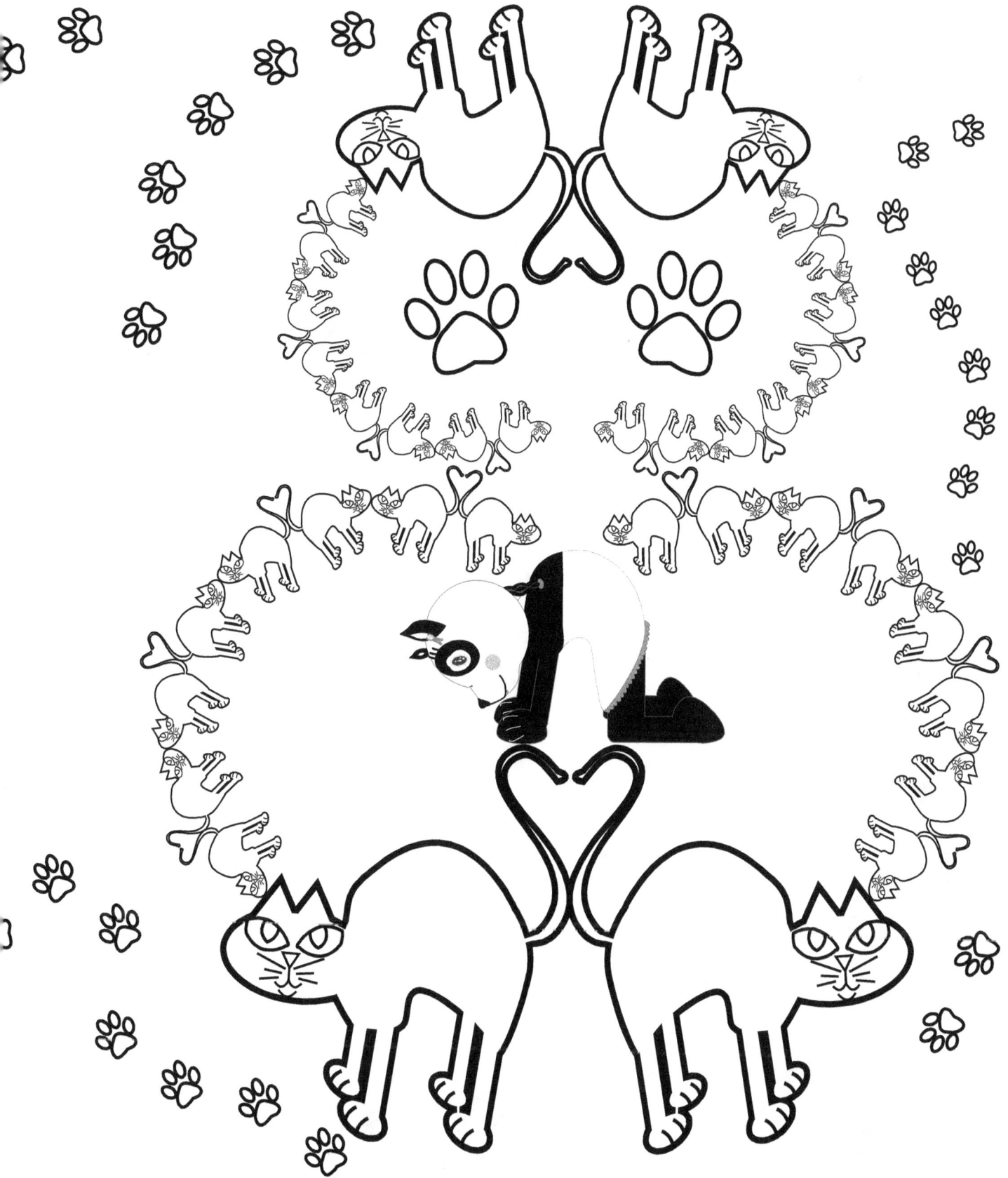

cat - gato

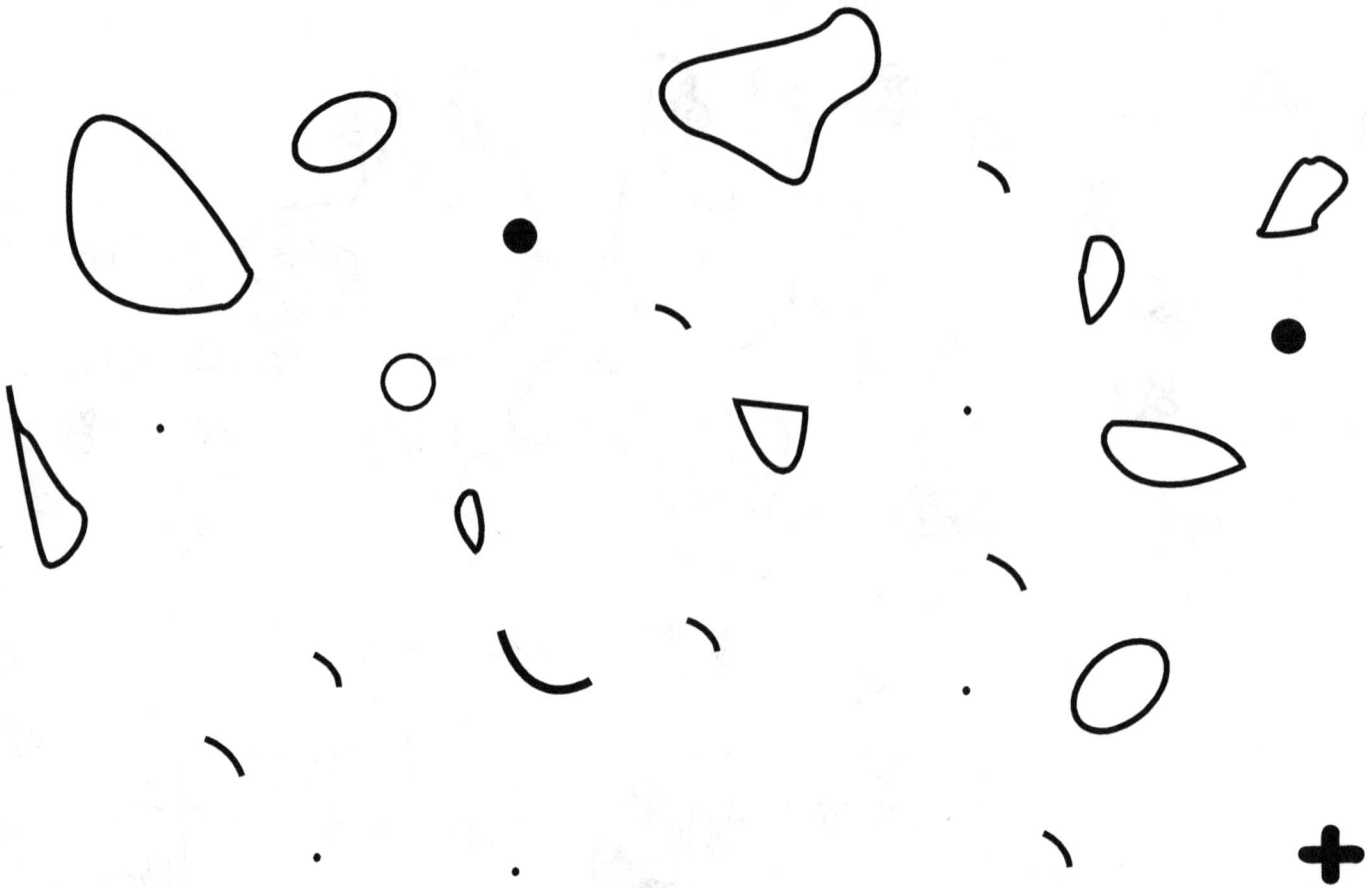

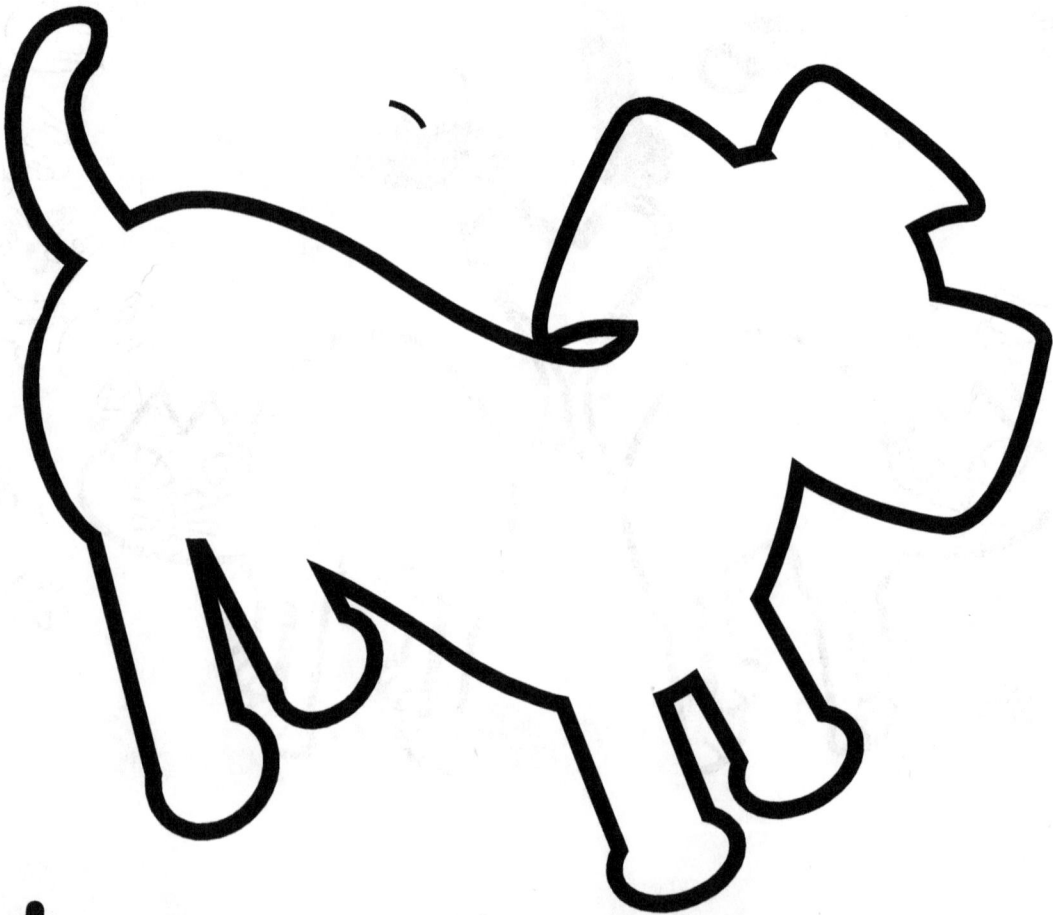

+

=

dog - perro

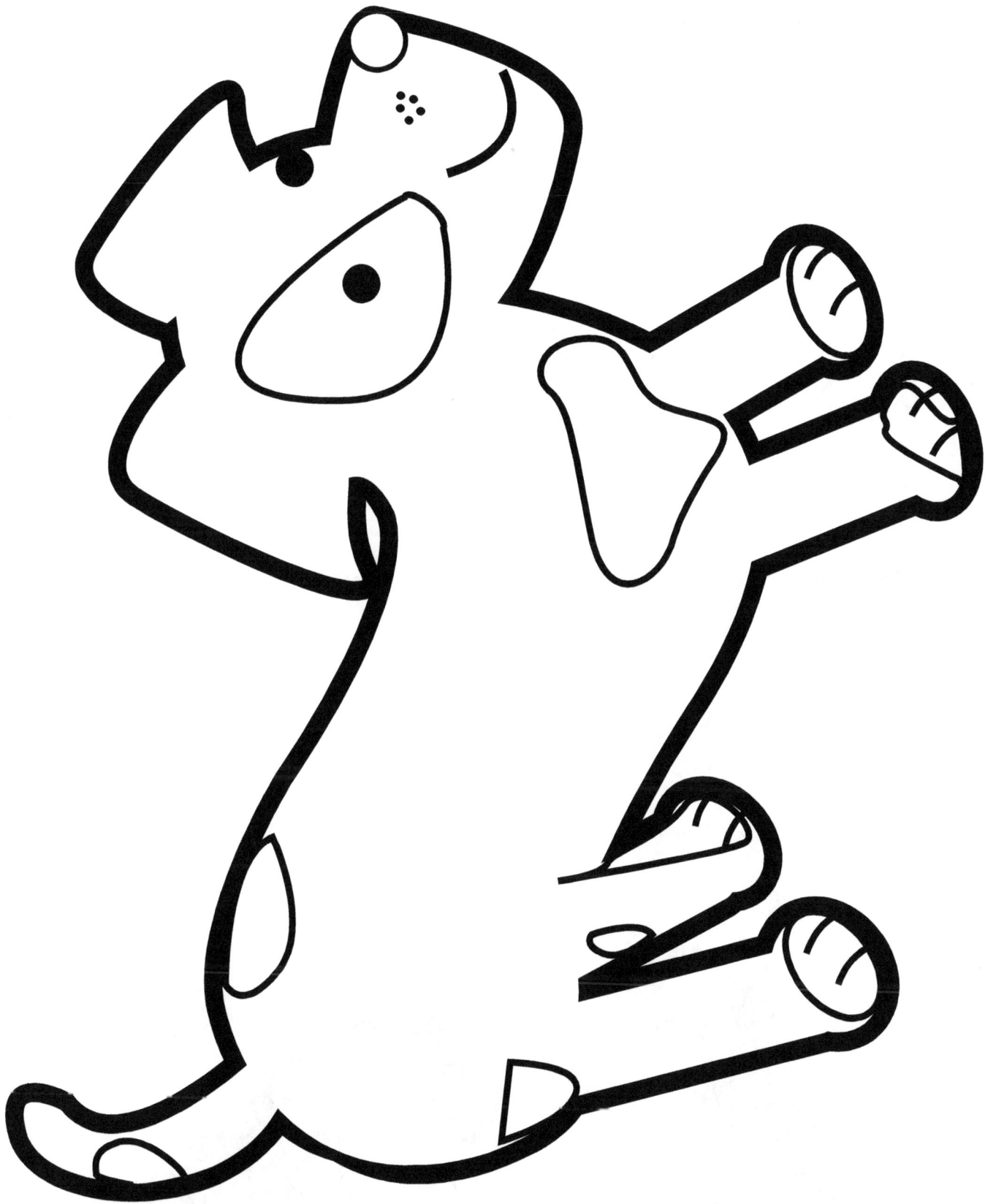

dog - perro

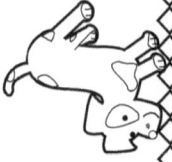

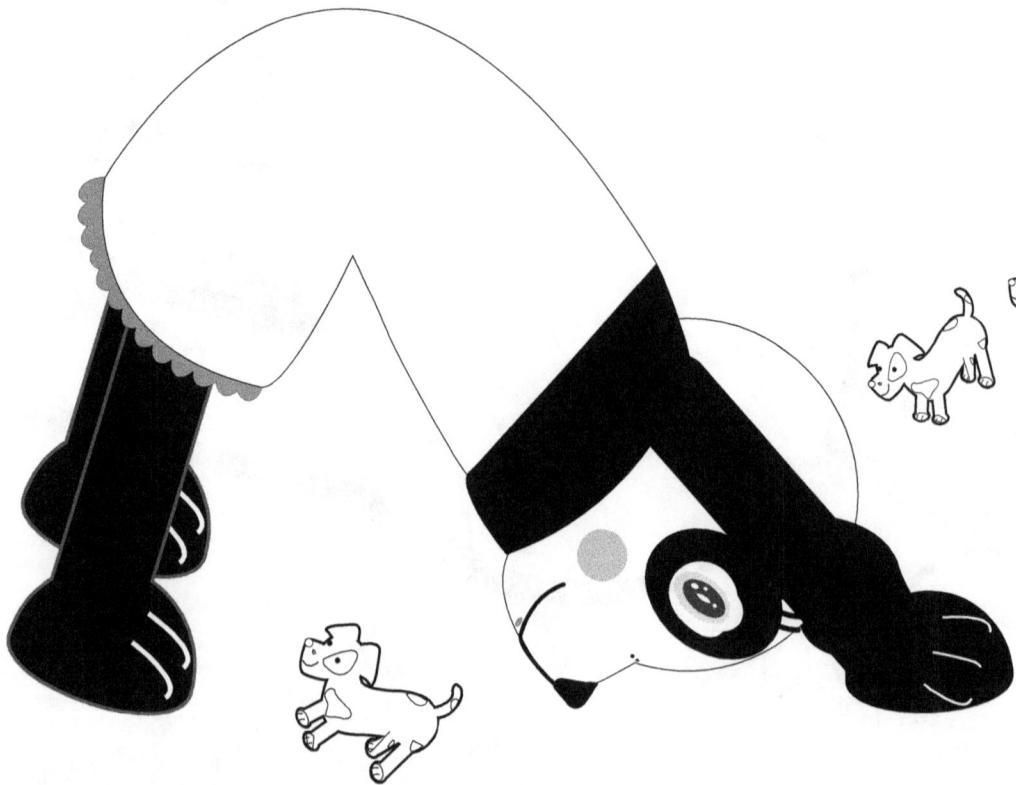

dog - perro

Happy Sachi's Yoga

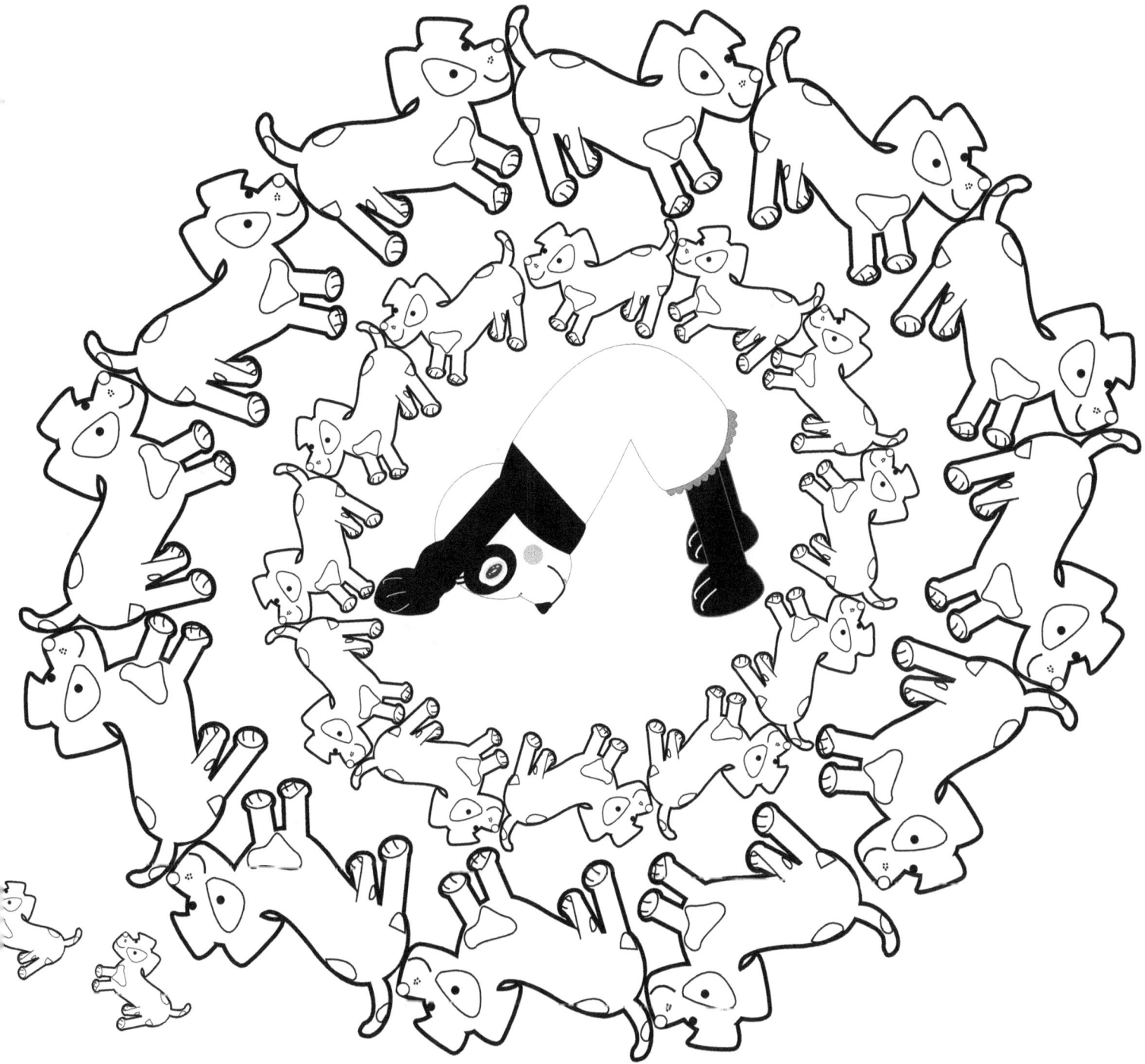

dog - perro

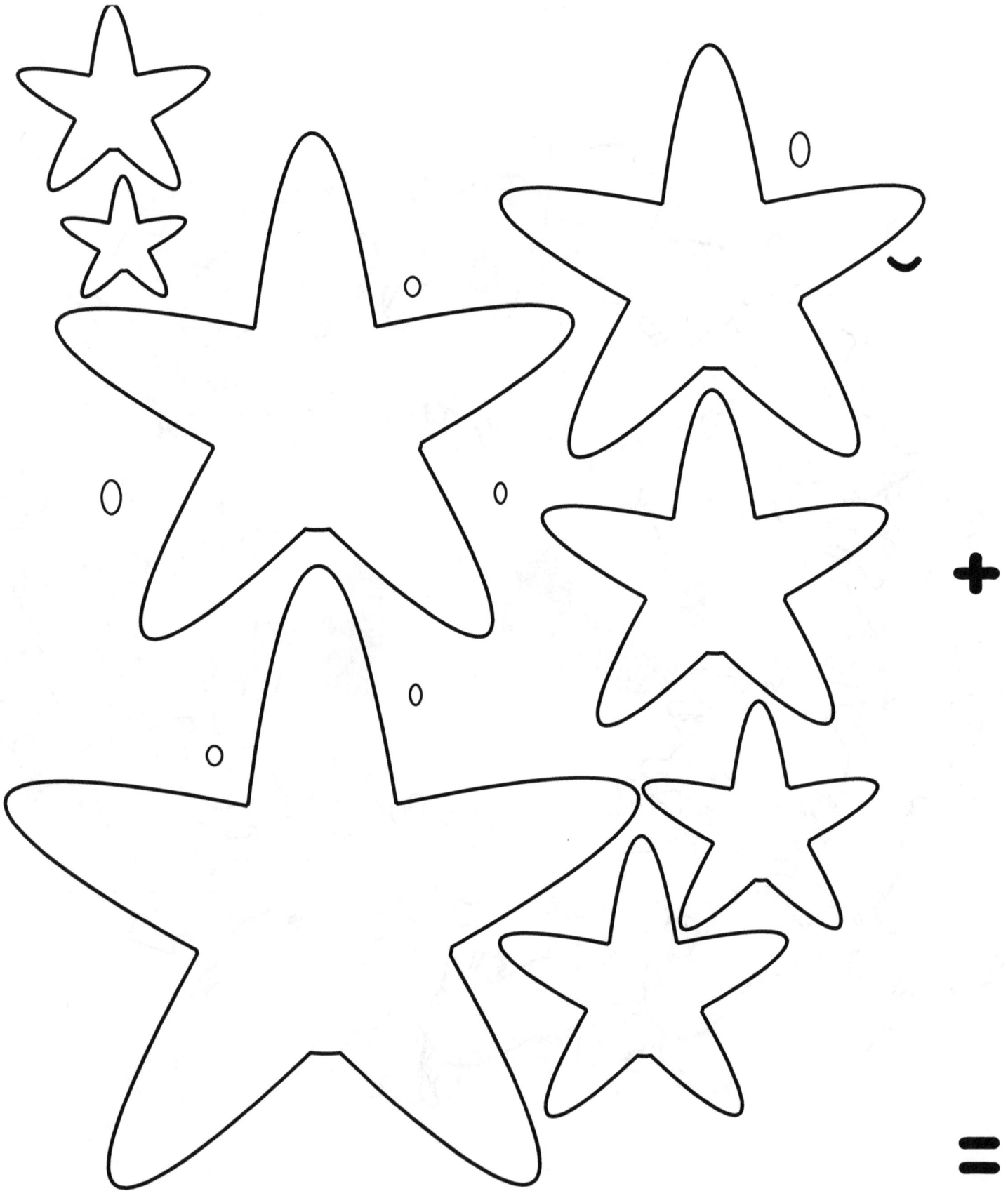

starfish - estrella de mar

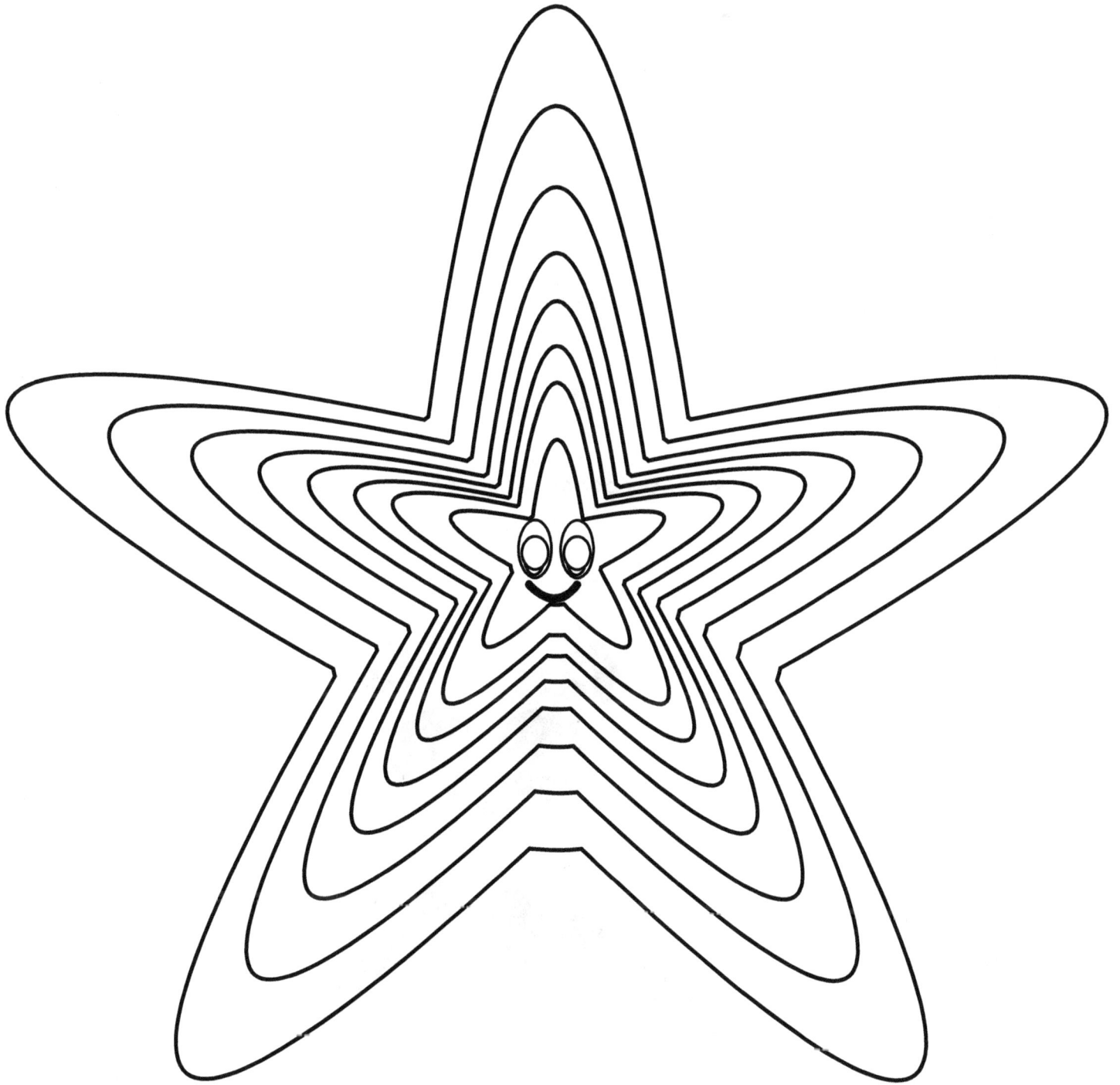

starfish - estrella de mar

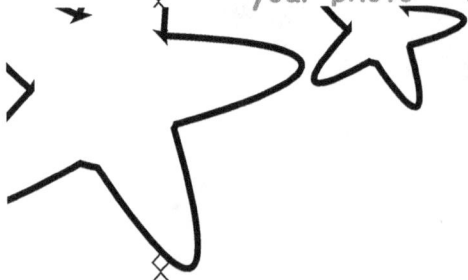

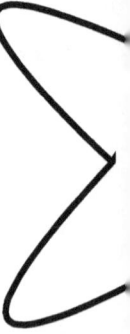

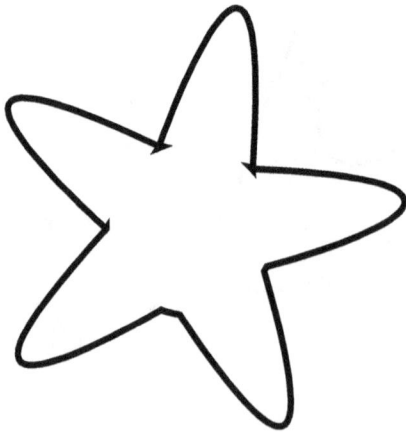

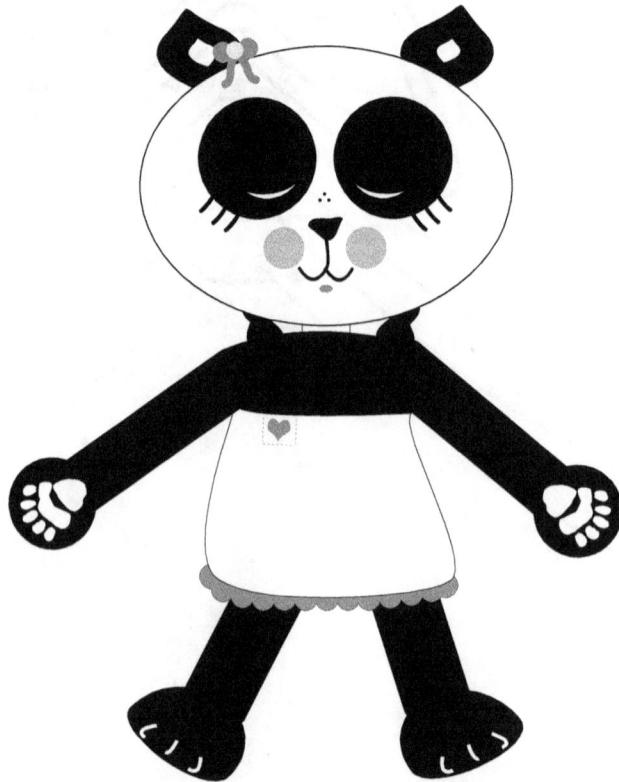

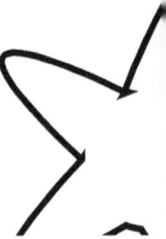

starfish - estrella de mar
Happy Sachi's Yoga

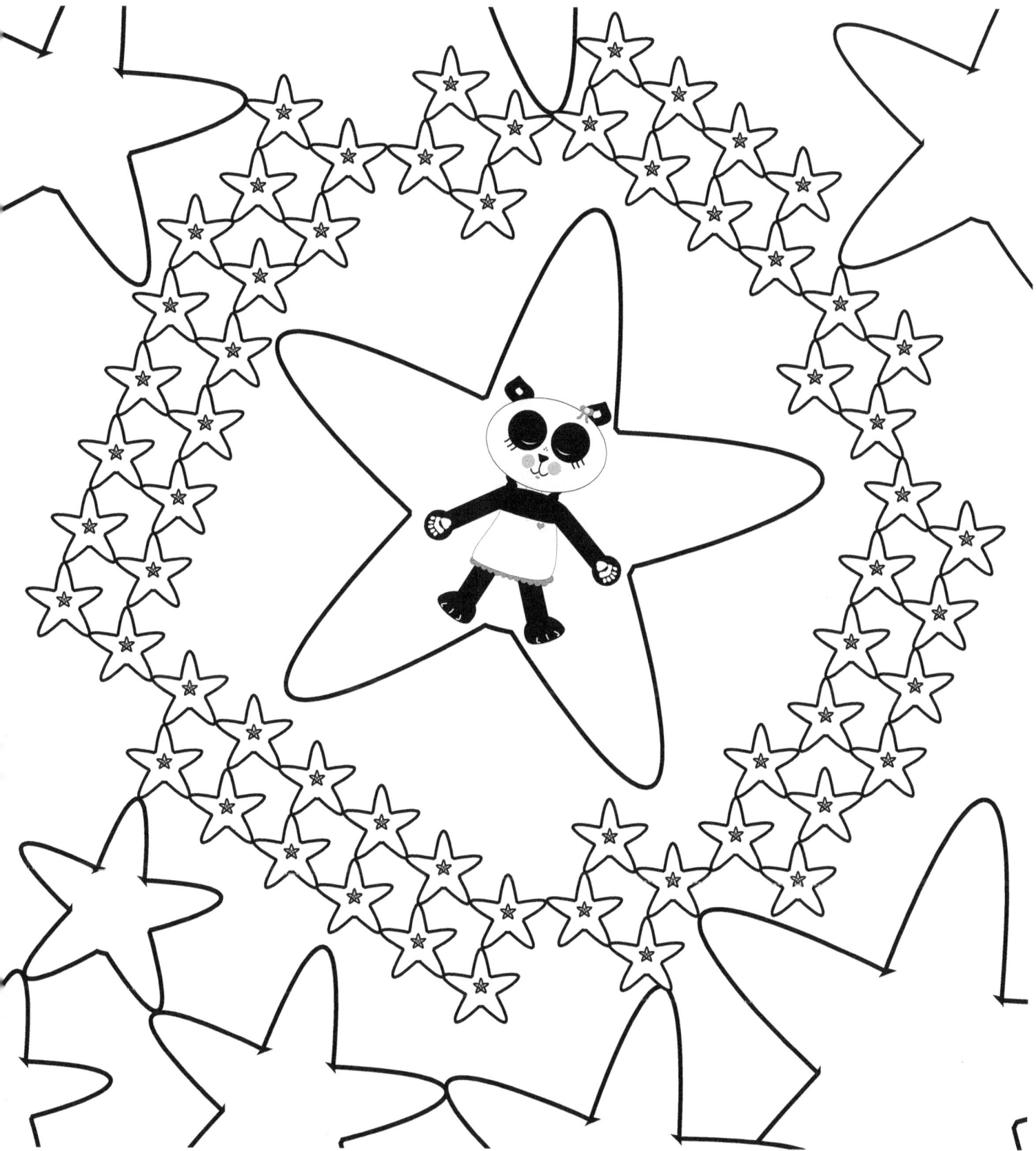

starfish - estrella de mar

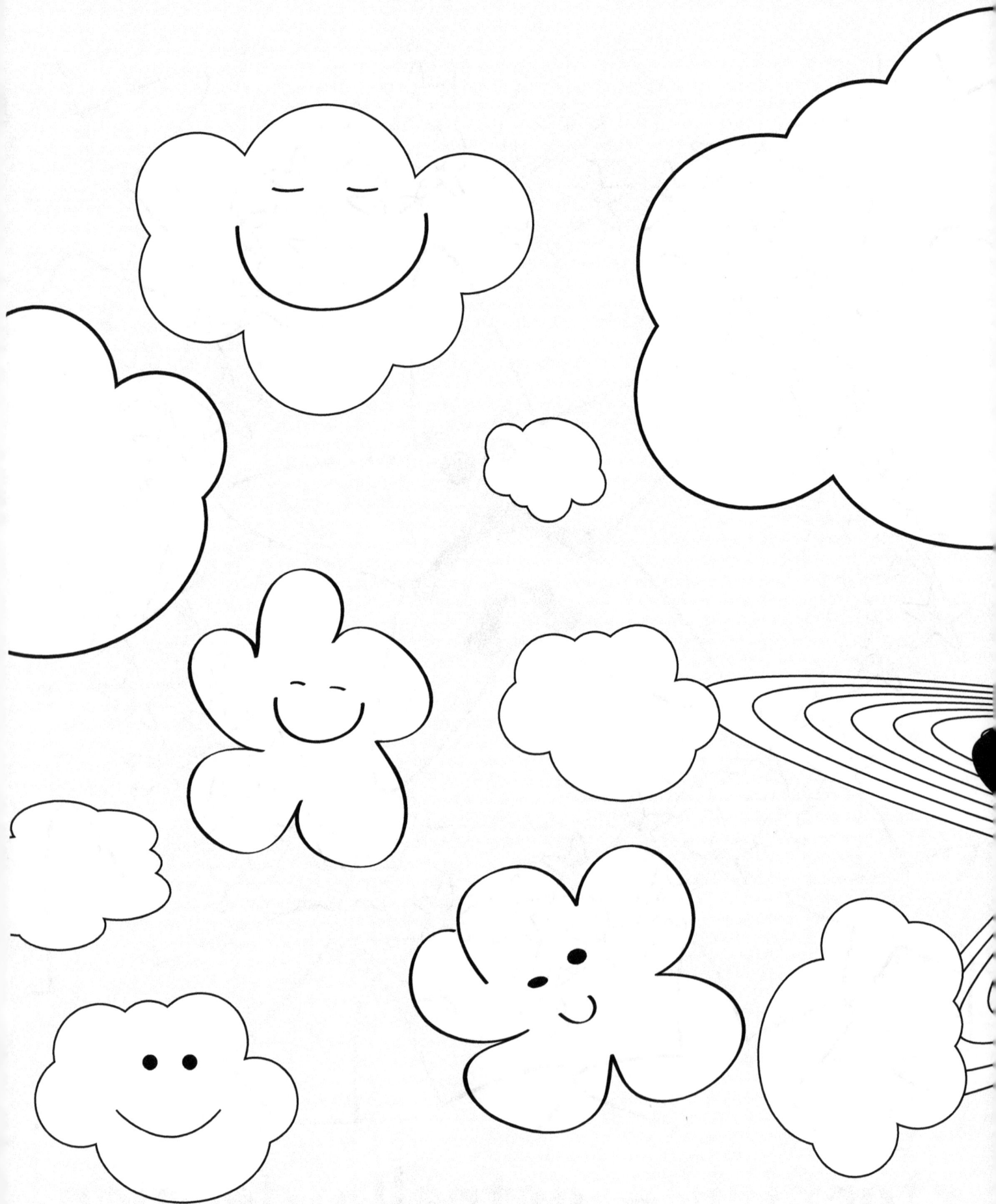

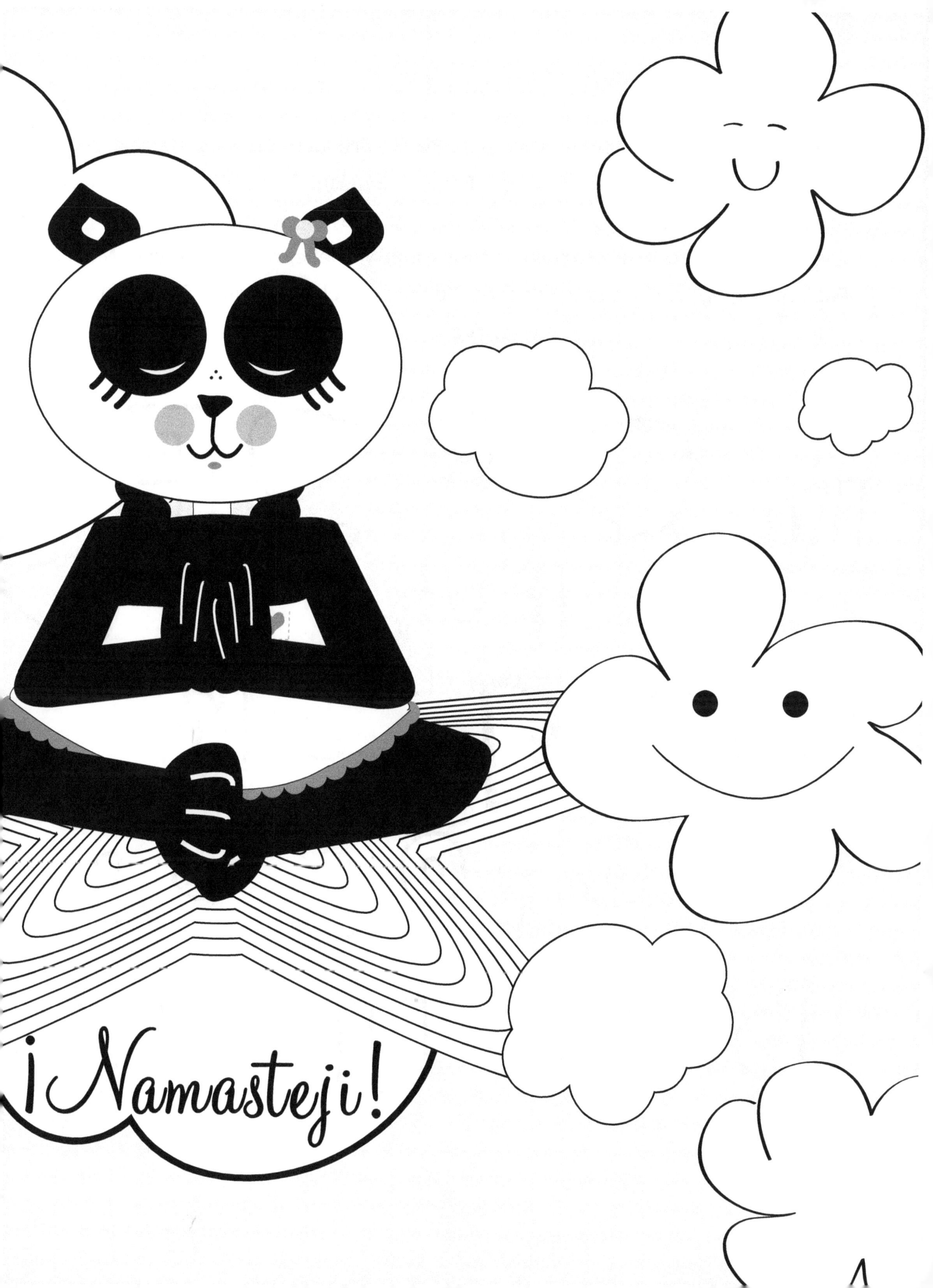

¡Namasteji!

Many Thanks - Muchas Gracias

Abu, Ajeet, Angel, Arjan, Audrey, Ben, Berta, Brendan, Camelia, Cecilia, Chen, Cindy, Dan, Daniel, David, Elisabeth, Francis, Ganesh, Gloria, Hari Kirin, Harumi, Hiroko, Hiroshi, Humberto, Irene, Ivan, Jai Hari, Jeymi, Joao, Jodi, Karla, Krishna, Lagrima, Luis, Liu, Maricruz, Marco, Mayumi, Michelle, Miyuki, Mireya, Mónica, Paulina, Rooni, Sandy, Sara, Sat Tara, Seibhang, Selene, Shabd, Shao Kun, Shuo, Valeria, Yuan, Ying, Xin.....

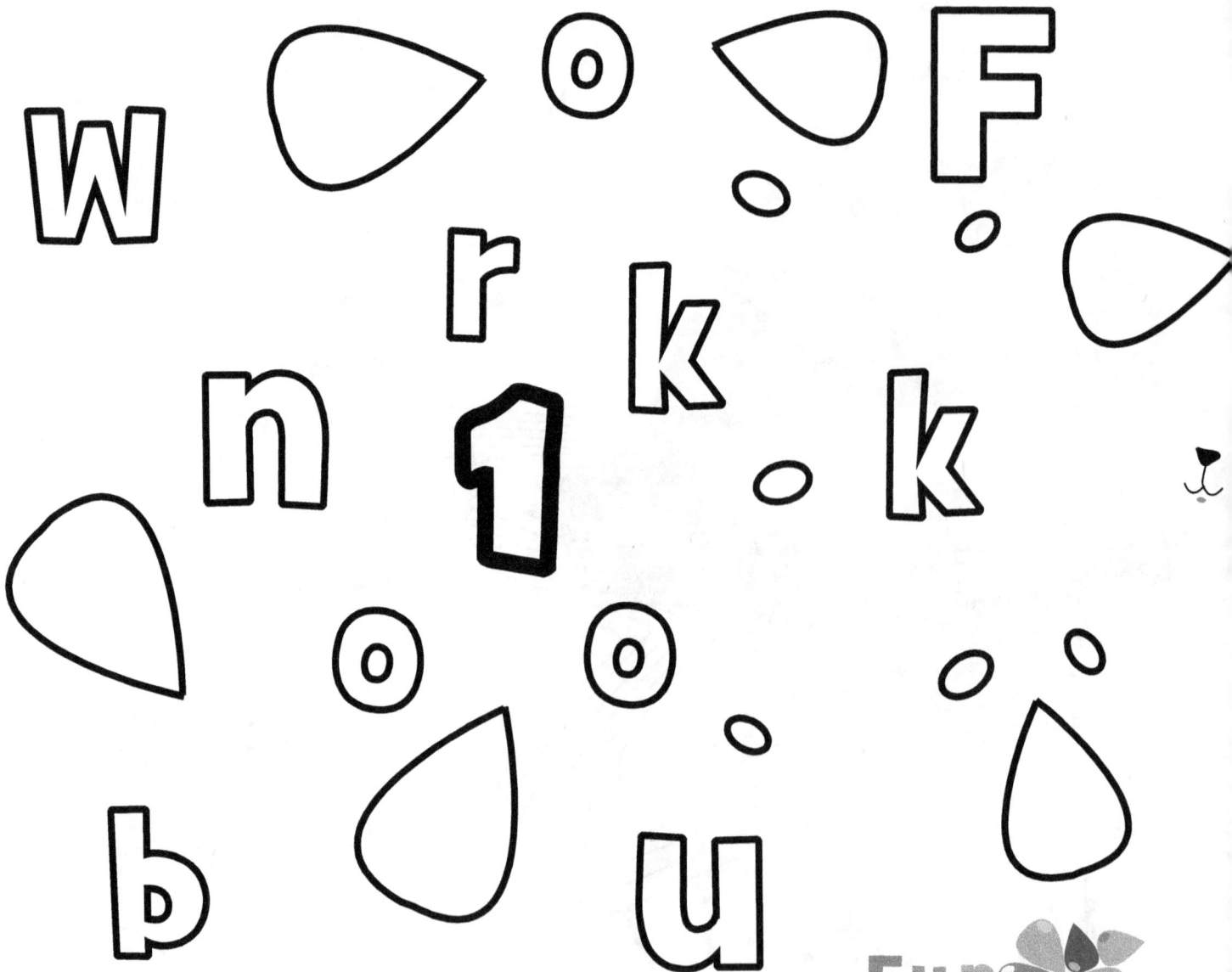

W o o F

w r k k

n 1 k

o o

b u